Evidence Based Medicine and Examination Skills: Translating Theory to Practice

Gastroenterology
Cardiology
Respiratory Medicine

Evidence Based Medicine and Examination Skills: Translating Theory to Practice

Gastroenterology
Cardiology
Respiratory Medicine

Neel Sharma

University Hospitals Birmingham NHS Foundation Trust,
Institute of Translational Medicine and
The Institute of Immunology and Immunotherapy, Birmingham, UK

World Scientific

NEW JERSEY · LONDON · SINGAPORE · BEIJING · SHANGHAI · HONG KONG · TAIPEI · CHENNAI · TOKYO

Published by

World Scientific Publishing Europe Ltd.

57 Shelton Street, Covent Garden, London WC2H 9HE
Head office: 5 Toh Tuck Link, Singapore 596224
USA office: 27 Warren Street, Suite 401-402, Hackensack, NJ 07601

Library of Congress Cataloging-in-Publication Data
Names: Sharma, Neel, author.
Title: Evidence based medicine and examination skills : translating theory to
    practice / by Neel Sharma.
Description: New Jersey : World Scientific, 2018. | Includes bibliographical
    references and index.
Identifiers: LCCN 2018044557 | ISBN 9781783269716 (hardcover : alk. paper)
Subjects: | MESH: Physical Examination--methods | Evidence-Based Medicine
Classification: LCC RC78.7.D53 | NLM WB 205 | DDC 616.07/54--dc23
LC record available at https://lccn.loc.gov/2018044557

British Library Cataloguing-in-Publication Data
A catalogue record for this book is available from the British Library.

For any available supplementary material, please visit
https://www.worldscientific.com/worldscibooks/10.1142/P1049#t=suppl

Typeset by Stallion Press
Email: enquiries@stallionpress.com

Contents

Part I
Gastroenterology

Motility Disorders: Achalasia

Aetiopathogenesis

Achalasia is associated with gross dilatation of the oesophagus and contraction of the lower oesophageal sphincter (LOS) as well as loss of myenteric neurons. Inhibitory neurons containing vasoactive intestinal polypeptide (VIP) and nitric oxide synthase (NOS) are lost, as well as excitatory neurons containing acetylcholine. The condition is associated with a significant inflammatory response with the existence of T lymphocytes and autoantibodies. Viral factors have been linked to the disease and include measles and varicella zoster. Achalasia can also occur secondary to malignancy, Chagas' disease, amyloidosis and sarcoidosis.

Symptoms

- Dysphagia for both liquids and solids
- Chest pain assumed to occur secondary to lactic acid production from fermentation of residual food debris
- Regurgitation secondary to retention of salvia and ingested food. Typically occurs in the recumbent position
- Weight loss

Signs

- Weight loss
- Possible chest signs secondary to aspiration

Differentials

- Angina
- Oesophageal cancer
- Oesophagitis
- Gastro-Oesophageal Reflux Disease (GORD)
- Scleroderma
- Oesophageal stricture

Investigations

An initial investigation of choice relies on a chest X-ray which typically shows an air fluid level. A barium swallow will demonstrate the classical appearances of a beak-like narrowing representing the non-relaxing LOS. Further investigations include a computed tomography (CT) scan which typically demonstrates a dilated oesophagus, and oesophageal manometry which will highlight the existence of an elevated basal LOS pressure. In some cases, however, LOS pressure may be normal or reduced. An endoscopy is useful in excluding secondary causes of achalasia such as carcinoma.

Management

Treatment comprises the use of calcium channel blockers, anti-cholinergics or nitrates which help to reduce the resting pressure of the LOS. Balloon dilatation has also been shown to reduce basal LOS pressure due to muscle fibre disruption. In some cases, patients may obtain relief from the use of endoscopic botulinum injection which helps to block cholinergic excitatory nerves in the LOS. From a surgical perspective, individuals may be able to undergo Heller myotomy which involves incision of the muscularis propria.

Diffuse Oesophageal Spasm

Aetiopathogenesis

Diffuse oesophageal spasm is thought to occur secondary to neural degeneration localised to nerve processes and inhibitory nerve dysfunction. Muscularis propria hypertrophy is also common.

Symptoms

- Chest pain
- Dysphagia
- Regurgitation

Signs

- Typically non-existent

Differentials

- Angina
- Oesophageal cancer
- Oesophagitis
- GORD
- Scleroderma
- Oesophageal stricture

Investigations

Barium swallow is the initial investigation of choice which demonstrates a corkscrew-like oesophagus. An oesophageal manometry can demonstrate the existence of swallow-induced contractions that are non-peristaltic in nature. A diagnosis is confirmed with >20% of wet swallows deteriorating into simultaneous onset contractions in the distal oesophagus.

Management

Treatment of diffuse oesophageal spasm often relies on anticholinergic agents, bougienage or botox-based therapies.

Gastro-Oesophageal Reflux Disease (GORD)

Aetiopathogenesis

One of the most common mechanisms for GORD is the occurrence of transient lower oesophageal sphincter relaxations (TLOSRs). During such activity, loss of the crural diaphragm occurs which impairs extrinsic sphincter function. Evidence also demonstrates that prolonged acid clearance is associated with worsening oesophagitis and a subsequent risk of Barrett's oesophagus. This can occur secondary to impaired peristalsis and hypotensive contractions. Increased abdominal pressure is also linked to GORD which explains why obese individuals or pregnant women are at risk from the condition. Following meals gastric juice occupies the top of the meal close to the cardia — commonly known as the acid pocket — which in patients with GORD, is located more proximally with respect to the squamocolumnar junction. GORD patients are also noted to experience increased hypersensitivity to acid.

Symptoms
- Heartburn commonly after lying supine or bending over
- Regurgitation
- Dysphagia
- Chest pain
- Cough or wheeze secondary to aspiration of gastric contents
- Hoarseness
- Nausea
- Vomiting

Signs

- Examination is typically unremarkable

Differentials

- Motility disorders e.g. achalasia
- Oesophageal cancer
- Oesophagitis
- Gastritis
- Peptic ulcer disease

Investigations

The primary investigation of choice is an upper gastrointestinal (GI) endoscopy. This allows for detection of oesophagitis, strictures and Barrett's oesophagus. The Los Angeles classification helps in the grading of reflux oesophagitis as follows:

- grade A oesophagitis: endoscopic abnormalities are restricted to one or more mucosal lesions with a maximum length of 5 mm.
- grade B oesophagitis: one or more mucosal breaks are present, with a maximum length of more than 5 mm but non-continuous across mucosal folds.
- grade C oesophagitis: mucosal breaks are continuous between at least two mucosal folds, but less than 75% of oesophageal circumference is involved.
- grade D oesophagitis: mucosal breaks encompass more than 75% of oesophageal circumference.

Manometry helps to determine LOS and oesophageal body function. It is undertaken in cases where there are persistence of symptoms whilst on treatment, recurrence of symptoms post-treatment, cessation as well as investigation of atypical symptoms. The use of a 24-hour pH probe is useful in cases where endoscopy is inconclusive. It helps to quantify GORD and allows for a correlation between reflux symptoms and episodes of reflux. Impedance monitoring is often used in conjunction with 24-hour pH monitoring helping to detect both acid and non-acid reflux.

Management

As per National Institute for Health and Care Excellence (NICE) guidelines, the treatment of GORD comprises proton pump inhibitors initially for up to two months followed by H2 receptor antagonists or prokinetic agents if there is an inadequate PPI response. Antireflux surgery is only considered in cases where an individual's quality of life is impaired.

Barrett's Oesophagus

Aetiopathogenesis

The primary factor for the development of Barrett's oesophagus is chronic GORD. Additional risk factors include an increasing body mass index (BMI) and central adiposity, which can lead to the formation of a hiatus hernia and increasing intragastric pressure, as well as smoking, an age > 50, male sex and Caucasian race. Protective factors include *Helicobacter pylori*, which reduces intragastric acid formation secondary to excess production of ammonia and parietal cell destruction. Genetic associations are noted and include dysfunction of the CDX2 gene.

Symptoms

- Heartburn
- Regurgitation
- Abdominal pain
- Chest pain
- Dysphagia

Signs

- Typically non-existent

Differentials

- GORD
- Oesophageal cancer
- Oesophageal motility disorders

- Peptic ulcer disease
- Hiatus hernia

Investigations

The gold standard investigation of choice is endoscopy and biopsy sampling, with note of the circumferential and maximum extent of the Barrett's segment. Histologically Barrett's oesophagus is determined by the presence of columnar-lined epithelium. Endoscopic ultrasound is often utilised to gain further understanding of disease staging in cases of suspected cancer.

Management

Treatment relies on acid suppression in the form of proton pump inhibitor (PPI) based therapy. Patients with evidence of low-grade dysplasia are typically monitored courtesy of repeat endoscopy and radiofrequency ablation. For high-grade dysplasia with visible lesions and early-stage Barrett's-associated adenocarcinoma, patients require endoscopic resection in the first instance. Patients with high-grade dysplasia or intramucosal cancer without visible lesions should be treated with ablation. Surgical intervention is appropriate for those patients with early adenocarcinoma which has extended into the submucosa.

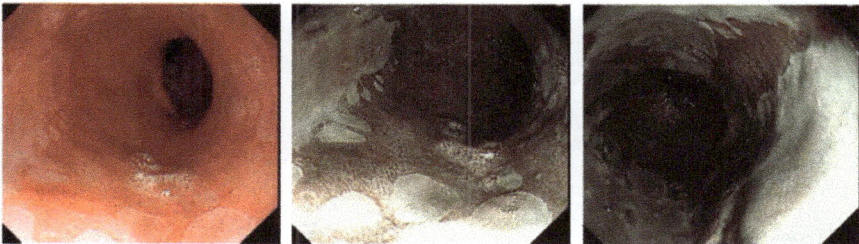

Fig. 1.   Evidence of Barrett's oesophagus at endoscopy

Oesophageal Perforation

Aetiopathogenesis

The occurrence of an oesophageal perforation or rupture is typically instrumental following an upper GI endoscopy. Therapeutic intervention such as oesophageal dilatation results in an increased risk of perforation. However, spontaneous rupture can also take place.

Symptoms

- Severe retrosternal chest pain, typically following retching/vomiting (Note such pain may radiate to the left shoulder or arm)
- Neck pain
- Dysphagia
- Facial swelling

Signs

- Tachycardia
- Tachypnoea
- Fever
- Subcutaneous emphysema
- Cyanosis

Differentials

- Abdominal compartment syndrome (ACS)
- Aortic dissection
- Peptic ulcer disease
- Pancreatitis

- PE
- Pneumothorax

Investigations

An erect chest X-ray helps to demonstrate evidence of infiltration or an effusion, typically seen on the left side. Mediastinal widening, a pneumomediastinum or subdiaphragmatic air may also be noted. A barium study can further aid diagnosis. More enhanced imaging may include a CT scan of the chest and abdomen. An upper GI endoscopy should be undertaken if imaging is inconclusive but suspicion remains high.

Management

Management relies on adequate fluid resuscitation and the use of intravenous antibiotics with immediate surgical intervention.

Hiatal Hernia

Aetiopathogenesis

Typically, the oesophagus enters the abdomen via the diaphragmatic hiatus, positioned at the level of the gastro-oesophageal junction. This hiatus is susceptible to visceral herniation due to pressure stress between the abdomen and chest. Two types of hiatal hernia exist: sliding which accounts for the majority and involves dilatation of the diaphragmatic hernia allowing the cardia of the stomach to herniate superiorly, and paraoesophageal hiatal hernia, where the herniated viscera herniates adjacent to the oesophagus. If there exists both sliding and paraoesophageal components, the hernia is regarded as mixed. Risk factors for the development of a hiatal hernia include age and obesity. Obesity has been shown to induce an increase in intra-abdominal pressure and hence hernia formation. Paraoesophageal hernias have been linked to gastro-oesophageal surgery, thoracoabdominal trauma and skeletal deformities.

Symptoms

- Heartburn
- Regurgitation
- Dysphagia
- Chest pain
- Abdominal pain, primarily epigastric in nature
- Nausea
- Vomiting

Signs

- Typically none

Differentials

- Oesophageal motility disorders e.g. achalasia
- Oesophagitis
- Coronary artery disease

Investigations

The investigation of choice is an upper GI endoscopy. Imaging in the form of a barium swallow is also useful.

Management

Treatment of GORD is essential in all cases with appropriate PPI-based therapy. Alternatives include H2 receptor antagonists and alginates. Surgical intervention in the form of a laparoscopic fundoplication aids in restoration of herniated organs within the abdominal cavity.

Peptic Ulcer Disease (PUD)

Aetiopathogenesis

PUD occurs secondary to an imbalance of gastric acid, pepsin and mucosal barrier function. Additional factors include smoking, alcohol, non-steroidal anti-inflammatory drugs (NSAIDs) and stress. *Helicobacter pylori* has been attributed to PUD as a result of decreased somatostatin production, increased gastrin and hence acid secretion. *H pylori* has been linked with inhibition of the neural antral inhibitory complex which stimulates parietal cells leading to increased acid production. There is also a resultant decrease in bicarbonate production as well as impaired acid clearance leading to inflammation and subsequently ulceration. The virulence factors associated with *H pylori* include CagA, VacA in the main as well as BabA and OipA. Inflammation occurs secondary to inflammatory cytokines such as interleukin 8 and interleukin 1β. Evidence also demonstrates a higher risk of PUD in patients with blood group O.

NSAIDs have been linked to ulcer formation as a result of prostaglandin synthesis inhibition. Neutrophil adherence is also key and allows for oxygen free radical release leading to protease release and impaired blood flow.

Symptoms

- Abdominal pain soon after meals in cases of gastric ulcer, and a few hours post with duodenal ulcers. Patients with the latter often experience pain at night
- Dyspepsia

- Heartburn
- Chest pain
- Haematemesis/melaena secondary to a bleeding ulcer
- Weight loss
- Dysphagia
- Vomiting

Signs
- Abdominal tenderness/rebound/guarding
- Melaena
- Haemodynamic instability in view of possible sepsis

Differentials
- Acute coronary syndrome
- Cholangitis
- Cholecystitis
- Diverticular disease
- Oesophagitis
- Gastritis
- Gastroenteritis
- GORD

Investigations
Routine blood investigations include a full blood count (FBC) (to exclude anaemia secondary to bleeding), urea and electrolyte (U and E) tests, liver function tests (LFTs) as well as serum amylase and lipase. The primary investigations include *Helicobacter* testing and an endoscopy. The former can be ascertained courtesy of a urease test i.e. Campylobacter-like organism (CLO) test or via faecal antigen testing. Although not routinely done, a serum gastrin level is worthwhile in cases of suspected Zollinger Ellison syndrome. In severe presentations, patients should undergo a chest X-ray to exclude evidence of perforation.

Management

Patients with peptic ulcer disease should have disease-provoking drugs such as NSAIDs stopped. If *H pylori*-positive, eradication should comprise a PPI, amoxicillin and clarithromycin or metronidazole and clarithromycin. A repeat endoscopy and retesting for *H pylori* is usually warranted in patients with gastric ulcers 6–8 weeks post-treatment. *H pylori*-negative patients should be treated with full dose PPI for 1–2 months. An inadequate response to PPI therapy requires the use of H2 receptor antagonists such as cimetidine.

Oesophageal and Gastric Cancer

Aetiopathogenesis

The risk factors for oesophageal cancer are dependent on pathological type. Squamous cell carcinoma (SCC) of the oesophagus is associated with smoking, alcohol and achalasia in the main. Oesophageal adeno-carcinoma is linked to prolonged GORD and Barrett's oesophagus in addition to obesity and poor dietary habits.

With regard to gastric cancer, intake of salt-enriched foods with minimal fruit and vegetables is associated with disease causation. The pathogen *Helicobacter pylori* is also linked with disease as is excess smoking and alcohol. Genetic factors play a part and include CDH1 mutations. Mismatch repair gene mutations are also linked with the phenomenon. Abnormal genomic function can also be seen secondary to the CpG island methylator phenotype.

Symptoms

- Weight loss
- Bleeding (haematemesis/melaena)
- Abdominal pain
- Hoarseness of voice
- Cough and additional chest-type symptoms
- Nausea/vomiting
- Dysphagia

Signs

- Lymphadenopathy (Virchow's node (left supraclavicular node enlargement in suspected gastric cancer)
- Hepatomegaly
- Dermatomyositis (gastric cancer-related)
- Acanthosis nigricans (gastric cancer-related)

Differentials

- Oesophagitis
- Gastritis
- PUD

Investigations

An endoscopy is the investigation of choice, particularly for patients over the age of 55 and presenting with alarm symptoms. Staging investigations include a CT scan of chest, abdomen and pelvis as well as endoscopic ultrasound/positron emission tomography (PET). Blood investigations of importance comprise a FBC (to exclude the existence of anaemia), U and E's and LFTs. Carcino embryonic antigen (CEA) and CA 19-9 tests are often raised in cases of gastric cancer but are typically non-specific.

Management

Endoscopic mucosal resection (EMR) and endoscopic submucosal dissection (ESD) can eradicate early gastro oesophageal (GO) cancer. Distal tumours are best treated by subtotal gastrectomy and proximal tumours by total gastrectomy. Stages II and III gastric cancer should undergo D2 lymphadenectomy.

Squamous cell oesophageal cancer should be treated by chemoradiation for localised proximal oesophageal disease. Localised squamous disease of the middle or lower third of the oesophagus should be treated by chemoradiotherapy alone or chemoradiotherapy plus surgery.

Oesophageal adenocarcinoma benefits from preoperative chemoradiation as compared to surgery alone. Typical chemotherapeutic agents include cisplatin and 5 Fluorouracil. Perioperative combination chemotherapy is the preferred choice for gastric cancer.

With regard to palliation for oesophageal cancer, external beam radiotherapy helps in relief of dysphagia, as does brachytherapy and chemotherapy (for example trastuzumab in combination with cisplatin/fluoropyrimidine for those with HER 2-positive oesophagogastric junctional adenocarcinoma. Tumours which are firm and stenosing resulting in significant dysphagia require a self-expanding stent. Argon plasma coagulation is useful in treating overgrowth above and below stents and in reducing bleeding from inoperable tumours. With regard to gastric cancer, palliative combination chemotherapy for locally advanced and metastatic disease is worthwhile (trastuzumab in combination with cisplatin/fluoropyrimidine should be considered for patients with HER 2-positive gastric tumours). It is important to note that in all cases, management relies on a multidisciplinary approach and patient involvement.

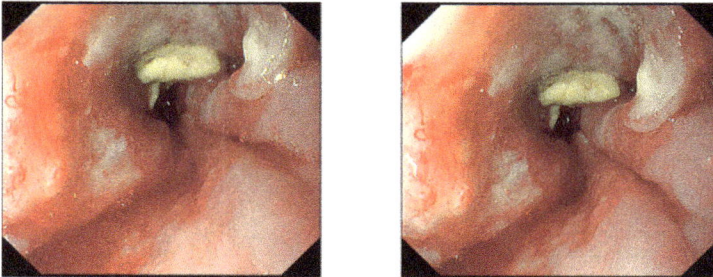

Fig. 2. Distal oesophagus tumour with evidence of food impaction

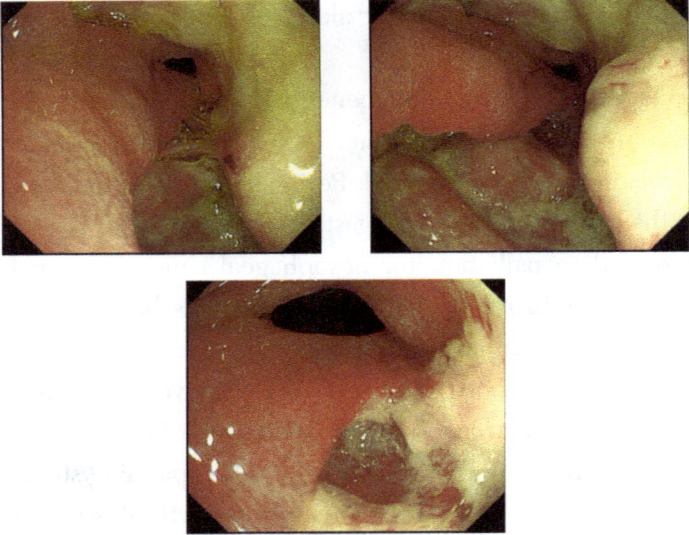

Fig. 3.   Gastric antrum tumour with ulceration

TOPIC

Upper GI Bleeding

Aetiopathogenesis

The causes and relative frequency of an upper GI bleed are detailed in Table 1.

Table 1: Major causes and relative frequency of upper GI bleeding

Cause of bleeding	Relative frequency (% of those in whom any abnormality was identified at endoscopy)
Peptic ulcer	44
Oesophagitis	28
Gastritis/erosions	26
Erosive duodenitis	15
Varices	13
Portal hypertensive gastropathy	7
Malignancy	5
Mallory Weiss tear	5
Vascular malformation	3

Symptoms

- Weakness
- Dizziness
- Fainting
- Coffee ground vomiting
- Black stools (melaena)
- Abdominal pain
- Indigestion
- Weight loss

Signs

- Haemodynamic instability e.g. tachycardia, hypotension, cool extremities
- Signs of chronic liver disease e.g. spider naevi, gynaecomastia, splenomegaly, ascites, asterixis
- Melaena
- Haematemesis
- Abdominal tenderness

Differentials

- Abdominal aortic aneurysm (AAA)
- Gastritis
- Oesophagitis
- PUD
- Gastric/oesophageal cancer

Investigations

Investigations of choice include a FBC, paying particular attention to the haemoglobin, platelet and white cell counts; U and E's; assessing for a rise in serum urea due to the presence of blood in the upper intestine; LFTs, coagulation profile, a group and save, and a crossmatch. Of course, the gold standard investigation is an endoscopy which provides an instant diagnosis and treatment intervention. An electrocardiogram (ECG) is useful to exclude a cardiac event, such as a myocardial infarction (MI) secondary to hypotension. Imaging is not often used but a chest X-ray may be required in cases of a suspected oesophageal perforation. In cases of continued bleeding and failure to cease via endoscopy, angiography is a useful alternative approach.

Management

According to NICE, patients with an upper GI bleed should undergo Blatchford scoring (see Table 2) at first assessment and Rockall scoring (see Table 3) post-endoscopy.

Table 2:   Blatchford Scoring

Haemoglobin	g/L
Blood urea nitrogen	mmol/L
Initial systolic blood pressure	mm Hg
Sex	❑ Male ❑ Female
Heart rate ≥ 100	+1 ▣ YES
Melaena present	+1 ▣ YES
Recent syncope	+2 ▣ YES
Hepatic disease history	+2 ▣ YES
Heart failure history	+2 ▣ YES

Table 3:   Rockall numerical risk scoring system

	Score				
Variable	0	1	2	3	
Age	< 60 years	60–79 years	≥ 80 years		
Shock	'no shock', SBP* ≥100 mm Hg, pulse <100 beats per minute	'tachycardia', SBP ≥100 mm Hg, pulse ≥100 beats per minute	'hypotension', SBP <100 mm Hg		Initial score criteria
Comorbidity	no major comorbidity		cardiac failure, ischaemic heart disease, any major comorbidity	renal failure, liver failure, disseminated malignancy	
Diagnosis	Mallory-Weiss tear, no lesion identified and no SRH	all other diagnoses	malignancy of upper GI tract		Additional criteria for full score
Major stigmata of recent haemorrhage (SRH)	none, or dark spot only		blood in upper GI tract, adherent clot, visible or spurting vessel		

Rockall score

Endoscopy should ideally be offered within the first 24 hours of admission. Table 4 shows the discharge and admission criteria for patients with upper GI bleeding.

Table 4:   Discharge and admission criteria for an upper GI bleed

Consider for discharge or non-admission with outpatient follow-up if:
- age < 60 years, and;
- no evidence of haemodynamic disturbance
  (systolic blood pressure $\geq$ 100 mm Hg, pulse < 100 beats per minute), and;
- no significant comorbidity
  (especially liver disease, cardiac disease, malignancy), and;
- not a current inpatient (or transfer), and;
- no witnessed haematemesis or haematochezia.

All such patients will have an initial Rockall score of 0. If aged > 60 years, the Rockall score becomes 1 and the patient should probably be admitted but considered for early discharge. Each patient must be assessed individually and clinical judgement should be used to guide these considerations.

Consider for admission and early endoscopy (and calculation of full Rockall score) if:
- age $\geq$ 60 years (all patients who are aged > 70 years should be admitted), or;
- witnessed haematemesis or haematochezia (suspected continued bleeding), or;
- haemodynamic disturbance (systolic blood pressure < 100 mm Hg, pulse $\geq$ 100 beats per minute), or;
- liver disease or known varices.

Table 5: Classification of hypovolaemic shock by blood loss in adults

	Class I	Class II	Class III	Class IV
Blood loss, volume (ml)	< 750	750–1,500	1,500–2,000	> 2,000
Blood loss (% of circulating blood)	0–15	15–30	30–40	> 40
Systolic blood pressure	No change	Normal	Reduced	Very reduced
Diastolic blood pressure	No change	Raised	Reduced	Very reduced/ unrecordable
Pulse (beats per minute)	Slight tachycardia	100–120	120 (thready)	> 120 (very thready)
Respiratory rate	Normal	Normal	Raised (> 20/min)	Raised (> 20/min)
Mental state	Alert, thirsty	Anxious or aggressive	Anxious, aggressive or drowsy	Drowsy, confused or unconscious

Adapted from Baskett PJF. ABC of major trauma: management of hypovolaemic shock. *BMJ.* 1990; 300: 1453–1457.

Table 5 shows shock classification by blood loss in adults suffering from an upper GI bleed. Fluid resuscitation is paramount in an upper GI bleed with red cell transfusion being considered after loss of 30% of circulating volume. Colloids or crystalloids can be used to achieve volume replacement prior to blood product administration.

Platelets should be transfused in those with a count of $< 50 \times 10^9/l$ and who are actively bleeding. Fresh frozen plasma is reserved for those with a fibrinogen level <1g/l or a prothrombin time/APTT >1.5 × normal. Patients on warfarin and who are actively bleeding require prothrombin complex.

Non-variceal bleeds should be treated with clips with or without adrenaline, thermal coagulation or fibrin. For continuous bleeding, one should repeat the endoscopy or explore the option of surgery. Proton pump inhibitors should be prescribed post-endoscopy in order to enhance blood coagulation. Patients with peptic ulcer bleeding should be assessed for *Helicobacter pylori* which should be eradicated in those testing positive. For variceal bleeds, patients should undergo band ligation followed by transjugular intrahepatic portosystemic shunt (TIPS) in case of failure. Balloon tamponade is recommended as a temporary treatment in uncontrolled variceal bleeds. It is important to note that terlipressin should be offered in cases of variceal bleeds. For gastric varices the optimum treatment of choice comprises N butyl 2 cyanoacrylate. A beta blocker should be prescribed as secondary prevention of an oesophageal variceal bleed. Patients with chronic liver disease presenting with an upper GI bleed should be treated with antibiotics as per microbiology input. Antibiotics of choice may include norfloxacin or ceftriaxone.

Patients on antiplatelet therapy at the time of a bleed should be discussed with appropriate specialists e.g. cardiology/neurology as to assess the risk and benefits of continuing such treatment. Other drugs of caution include selective serotonin reuptake inhibitors (SSRIs), anticoagulants and steroids.

Acute Diarrhoea

Aetiopathogenesis

In acute cases of diarrhoea, several bacterial agents can lead to symptoms. *E coli* (EC) has been attributed to the occurrence of traveller's diarrhoea with bloody diarrhoea noted with enteroinvasive (EIEC) and enterohaemorrhagic (EHEC) forms. Enterohaemorrhagic *E coli* is commonly associated with ground beef. *Campylobacter* is another bacterial agent associated with watery diarrhoea with poultry an important source. *Shigella* is a common cause of diarrhoea in children with Sd1 leading to significant and often fatal occurrences of bloody stool formation. *Vibrio cholerae* leads to watery mucus-filled stool with co-existing vomiting. *Salmonella* is associated with watery or blood- enriched diarrhoea with associated enteric fever and is a common contaminant of eggs.

Viral-based agents of acute diarrhoea include rotavirus and norovirus in the main which are linked to non-bloody diarrhoea and vomiting. Parasitic agents are also worth a mention and include *Giardia*, associated with malodorous greasy stools; *Cryptosporidium*, linked to watery diarrhoea and abdominal cramps; and *Entamoeba histolytica*, associated with abdominal cramps and bloody/watery diarrhoea in the main.

Symptoms

Apart from the obvious (!), additional symptoms can include:
- Vomiting
- Flatulence
- Blood and mucus PR

Signs

- Dehydration, namely sunken eyes, reduced tissue turgor, delayed capillary refill, abdominal pain/cramps
- Borborygmi
- Muscle wasting

Differentials

- Appendicitis
- Inflammatory bowel disease
- Irritable bowel syndrome
- Thyroid dysfunction

Investigations

Investigations rely on a FBC (to exclude infection), U and E's (in view of dehydration), and a C-reactive protein (CRP) including stool cultures for microscopy culture & sensitivity, Ova Cysts and Parasites and *C difficile*. Imaging is generally not required but may include an abdominal X-ray in the first instance. Prolonged diarrhoea may require colonoscopy and biopsy.

Management

Management of acute diarrhoea relies on appropriate fluid resuscitation in the first instance, either through oral rehydration therapy or intravenous fluids. Anti-motility agents such as loperamide is recommended in mild to moderate non-inflammatory cases of traveller's diarrhoea. Infective cases, however, are treated depending on cause; note examples highlighted below:

- Cholera   Doxycycline/tetracycline
- Shigella   Ciprofloxacin
- Amoebiasis   Metronidazole
- Giardiasis   Metronidazole
- Campylobacter   Azithromycin

Chronic Diarrhoea

Aetiopathogenesis

The aetiopathogenesis of chronic diarrhoea in the developed world seems to lie in accordance with irritable bowel syndrome (IBS), inflammatory bowel disease (IBD), malabsorption syndrome, chronic infection and idiopathic secretory diarrhoea. In developing nations, attributes of chronic diarrhoea comprise bacterial and parasitic-based infections.

Symptoms and signs are much the same as acute diarrhoea. It goes without saying that the underlying cause can determine presentation.

Differentials

- Colonic cancer
- IBD
- Coeliac disease
- Bile salt malabsorption
- Bacterial overgrowth
- Pancreatitis
- Thyroid dysfunction

Investigations

Investigations comprise a FBC, LFTs, tests for serum calcium and B12/folate/ferritin, a thyroid function test (TFT) and coeliac serology in the first instance. Endoscopy and biopsy are useful as well as a barium follow through. To exclude possible pancreatic dysfunction, one can consider the use of a CT scan or faecal elastase in addition to an endoscopic retrograde cholangio pancreatography (ERCP)/magnetic resonance cholangio pancreatography (MRCP). Stools should be weighed for a 24–72 hour period with osmolality assessment as well as a laxative screen. Additional tests of choice include the glucose hydrogen breath test/jejunal aspirate and culture to exclude bacterial overgrowth as well as serum gastrin (to exclude a gastrinoma), a vasoactive intestinal polypeptide test (to exclude a VIPoma) and urinary 5-Hydroxyindoleacetic acid (to determine the existence of carcinoid tumours). For suspected small bowel disease, it is advised that patients undergo barium follow through studies or Tc HMPAO scanning. Bile acid malabsorption can be excluded courtesy of SeHCAT testing.

Management

Treatment of chronic diarrhoea relies on management of the underlying cause in the first instance. For example, infectious causes rely on antibiotics as per microbiology. Certain foods should be eliminated as should sorbitol which can exacerbate the problem.

Medications of choice include bismuth, bile acid binding agents such as cholestyramine in the case of bile salt malabsorption, a high fibre diet, anti-diarrhoeal medication such as loperamide and in cases of carcinoid, octreotide.

Faecal Incontinence

Aetiopathogenesis

In order to appreciate the occurrence of faecal incontinence, one must appreciate the normal anal sphincter complex, which comprises the internal and external anal sphincter as well as the puborectalis muscle, both of which are highly innervated. Both the external anal sphincter and puborectalis muscle are responsible for voluntary sphincter contraction, whereas the internal anal sphincter is involuntary in nature. Disruption to this complex is responsible for the occurrence of faecal incontinence. Causes may be congenital such as an imperforate anus or meningocele, anatomical due to obstetric or rectal surgery, neurological such as multiple sclerosis, stroke and dementia or secondary to conditions such as diabetes, IBD, malabsorption, malignancy, rectal prolapse or psychiatric disturbance.

Symptoms
- Faecal urgency
- Anal pruritus
- Liquid/solid stool
- Flatus

Signs
- Perineal deformity secondary to surgery
- Anal gaping suggestive of prolapse
- PR examination demonstrating impaction/diminished anal tone/ sensation

Differentials

- Colorectal cancer
- Cauda equina syndrome
- IBD
- Acute/chronic diarrhoea

Investigations

Imaging is an essential investigative tool in the diagnosis of faecal incontinence. Endoanal ultrasound and magnetic resonance imaging (MRI) provide appropriate structural detail. Assessment of function comes courtesy of manometry providing analysis of the internal and external anal sphincter and rectal sensation. Pudendal nerve terminal motor latency (PNTML) testing is also employed to determine any obvious pudendal neuropathy leading to faecal incontinence. Defecography, where a barium paste is emptied under fluoroscopy, can be utilised to assess for any pelvic floor pathology contributing to faecal incontinence.

Management

Medical therapy in the first instance is essential comprising increased fibre and bowel habit training. Idiopathic diarrhoea is best managed with medication such as loperamide and bulking agents such as psyllium. Biofeedback approaches are also instigated to aid in sphincter muscle contraction following rectal distension, sensory training allowing for smaller volumes of rectal distension to be recognised and strength training of the sphincter muscle without rectal distension. Surgical intervention is employed for sphincter defects such as a sphincteroplasty, where the damaged sphincter is dissected back to healthier muscle. Faecal diversion is also an alternative through stoma formation. Innovative options comprise graciloplasty which involves transposition of the gracilis muscle with electrical stimulation as well as artificial anal sphincters and sacral nerve stimulation.

TOPIC

Constipation

Aetiopathogenesis

Constipation occurs secondary to organic and functional causes. Numerous factors exist and include a low fibre diet, dementia, depression and limited fluid intake, metabolic dysfunction such as diabetes, hypercalcaemia, hypokalaemia and hypothyroidism, neurological causes such as Parkinson's disease, multiple sclerosis and spinal cord dysfunction, drugs such as aluminium-containing antacids, iron, antidepressants, anti-cholinergics and opiates, and anorectal abnormalities such as fissures, fistulae and abscesses.

Symptoms

- Abdominal bloating
- Pain
- Rectal bleeding
- Diarrhoea secondary to overflow
- Weight loss

The ROME diagnostic criteria is a useful aid for symptom evaluation, requiring at least two or more of the following symptoms:

- Straining during at least 25% of defecations
- Lumpy or hard stools in at least 25% of defecations
- Sensation of incomplete evacuations for at least 25% of defecations
- Sensation of anorectal obstruction/blockage for at least 25% of defecations
- Manual manoeuvres to facilitate at least 25% of defecations
- Fewer than three bowel movements a week

Signs

- Rectal assessment with possible evidence of fissures, masses, impacted stool, rectal prolapse
- Evidence of contributing pathology e.g. signs of hypothyroidism, diabetes, neurological dysfunction

Differentials

- Anxiety
- Colon cancer
- IBD
- Hypothyroidism
- Hypopituitarism
- Irritable bowel syndrome

Investigations

Initial blood investigations are key and include a FBC to exclude anaemia, TFT's to exclude hypothyroidism and an electrolyte screen in view of potential metabolic abnormalities. Imaging is essential and comprises an abdominal X-ray in the first instance with the utilisation of a CT/MRI/barium study. For those patients suspected of motility disorders, a colonic transit study is typically instigated. A lower GI endoscopy can also be undertaken but it is important to be mindful of potential perforation. Anorectal manometry allows for sphincter analysis as well as pressure determination. Additional investigations may include a balloon expulsion test to help exclude defecation disorders.

Management

Management of constipation is classically cause-dependent. For example, anal fissures benefit by applying glyceryl trinitrate (GTN) topically. A high fibre diet, hydration, physical activity and enemas/laxatives are essential in the management of constipation in general, with stimulant-based laxatives particularly useful in cases of slow transit constipation. Biofeedback therapies have been trialled in cases of obstructive defecation to aid patients in pelvic floor relaxation.

TOPIC

Coeliac Disease

Aetiopathogenesis

Coeliac disease is associated with prolonged inflammation of the small bowel secondary to gluten. The proteins gliadin and glutenin within gluten are both toxic and immunogenic. Genetic associations have been linked with HLA DQ2 and DQ8. Additional susceptibility has been linked with COELIAC2 (5q31–33), 3 (2q33) and 4 (19p13.1) as well as 4q27. Infectious agents have been associated with coeliac disease including rotavirus. With regard to pathogenesis, gluten peptides are transported across the intestinal epithelium which are then presented to CD4 + T cells by dendritic cells following deamidation of gluten by tissue transglutaminase. Once activated, CD4 + T cells produce inflammatory cytokines inducing a Th1 response courtesy of IFN γ. This subsequently leads to the release of matrix metalloproteinases (MMPs) which leads to the breakdown of the extracellular matrix and basement membrane as well as increased cytotoxicity of intraepithelial lymphocytes (IELs). This results in the apoptotic death of enterocytes. Finally the production of Th 2 cytokines leads to the activation of B cells, which produce antigliadin and anti-tissue transglutaminase antibodies. The latter is associated with enterocyte damage.

Symptoms

- Diarrhoea secondary to malabsorption
- Flatulence
- Weight loss
- Fatigue

- Abdominal bloating or cramps
- Bone pain due to osteopenia/osteoporosis due to vitamin D deficiency and defective calcium transport
- Neurological symptoms such as motor weakness, sensory loss, ataxia, fits due to hypocalcaemia
- Skin rash

Signs

- Abdominal bloating
- Peripheral oedema due to hypoalbuminaemia
- Ecchymoses secondary to vitamin K malabsorption
- Glossitis
- Dermatitis herpetiformis
- Peripheral neuropathy
- Chvostek's or Trousseau's sign

Differentials

- Bacterial overgrowth
- IBD
- Gastroenteritis
- IBS
- Hypothyroidism

Investigations

Investigations comprise the use of tissue transglutaminase antibodies and endomysial antibodies. Patients should undergo screening for IgA levels and if deficient, the IgG isotype of autoantibodies should be measured. A tissue diagnosis is important and relies on the use of a duodenal biopsy to determine the degree of villous atrophy. If symptoms persist after six months, a repeat biopsy is advisable. In addition, patients should undergo measurement of bone density via dual-energy X-ray absorptiometry (DEXA). Blood investigations rely on the exclusion of hypokalaemia, hypocalcaemia and hypomagnesaemia as well as a low serum albumin. Patients should be screened for iron, folate and B12 deficiency as well as assessment of prothrombin time which may be prolonged due to vitamin K malabsorption.

Management

Management comprises the use of a gluten-free diet with avoidance of wheat, rye and barley. Oats are typically safe as long as they are truly free from wheat contamination. In addition, all individuals with coeliac disease should consume 1,500 mg calcium per day.

Irritable Bowel Syndrome (IBS)

Aetiopathogenesis

Studies focusing on the pathogenesis of IBS suggest one particular factor of abnormal motility, where high amplitude contractions serve to exist in those presenting with abdominal pain and diarrhoea. However, motility abnormalities in the main are not uniform. In addition, another factor of interest is visceral hypersensitivity which is demonstrated in IBS-affected patients. In post-infectious cases of IBS, there is evidence of increased mast cells and lymphocytes. Autonomic dysfunction exists and can take place in the form of cardiovagal dysfunction in those with constipation-predominant symptoms and sympathetic adrenergic dysfunction in those with diarrhoea. Research on brain imaging has also indicated that abnormal visceral afferent processing by the brain is an occurrence in IBS individuals. And finally it is important to appreciate the intensity of psychosocial factors with stress, underlying psychiatric disorders and significant life events inducing IBS-based symptoms.

Symptoms

Symptoms of IBS rely on the ROME III criteria depicted in Table 6.

Table 6:   ROME III criteria for IBS

Diagnostic criterion*
Recurrent abdominal pain or discomfort** at least 3 days/month in the last 3 months associated with two or more of the following:
1. Improvement with defecation
2. Onset associated with a change in frequency of stool
3. Onset associated with a change in form (appearance) of stool

*Criterion fulfilled for the last 3 months with symptom onset at least 6 months prior to diagnosis
** "Discomfort" means an uncomfortable sensation not described as pain.
In pathophysiology research and clinical trials, a pain/discomfort frequency of at least 2 days a week during screening evaluation is recommended for subject eligibility.

Signs

- Typically non-existent. However, sigmoid tenderness on palpation has been reported

Differentials

- Coeliac disease
- Gastroenteritis
- IBD
- Thyroid dysfunction
- Lactose intolerance
- Bacterial overgrowth
- Bile salt malabsorption
- Colon cancer

Investigations

The diagnosis of IBS is based on exclusion. Investigations comprise a FBC (for the exclusion of anaemia and infection), erythrocyte sedimentation rate (ESR) and CRP, U and E's (to determine the degree of dehydration in those with significant diarrhoea) and TFTs, in addition to a coeliac screen for tissue transglutaminase antibodies. A lactose breath hydrogen test is recommended as well as a SeHCAT test in cases of large diarrhoeal volumes. As IBS is a functional diagnosis, patients require a CT and colonoscopy to exclude organic pathology. Stool should be sent for MC and S, ova, cysts and parasite and *C. difficile*. Recommendations also exist for the undertaking of psychological investigation through the Hospital Anxiety and Depression Scale (HADS) or PHQ15.

Management

The management of IBS relies on a multitude of intervention. From a dietary perspective, fibre intake should be assessed and increased/decreased accordingly. It is also recommended that a trial of exclusion of wheat, bran or lactose should occur and dietary modification based on particular intolerances. Psychological treatments are also relevant and include relaxation therapy, cognitive behavioral therapy (CBT), hypnotherapy and interpersonal therapy. Depending on symptomatology, the following agents may be of value:

- Pain   Antispasmodics/tricyclic antidepressants
- Diarrhoea   Loperamide
- Constipation Ispaghula

Bloating-type symptoms may benefit from probiotics, polyethylene glycols and antispasmodics.

Whipple's Disease

Aetiopathogenesis

The primary factor associated with Whipple's disease is the pathogen *Tropheryma whipplei* which is known to replicate within macrophages, leading to apoptosis of host cells and further bacterial spread. It is assumed that an array of cytokines, interleukin 16 being one example, are responsible for such an occurrence. The overall inflammatory response that ensues results in multi-systemic pathology. One observes a reduction in Th1 cells and an increased Th2 cell population.

Symptoms

- Diarrhoea secondary to malabsorption
- Joint pain
- Fever
- Weight loss
- Cardiac and neurological-related symptomatology

Signs

- Joint swelling
- Malabsorption stigmata e.g. cachexia, abdominal distension, cheilitis, gingivitis
- Neurological signs e.g. ataxia, clonus, supranuclear ophthalmoplegia
- Cardiac signs e.g. endocarditis/pericarditis
- Respiratory manifestations e.g. pleural effusion, interstitial lung disease
- Hyperpigmentation

Differentials

- Coeliac disease
- Tropical sprue

Investigations

A valuable diagnostic test for Whipple's disease is determining the presence of *T whipplei*. For GI-related manifestations, the diagnostic test of choice is duodenal jejunal biopsies for periodic acid–Schiff-positive foamy macrophages. Blood investigations demonstrate a raised ESR in addition to low iron and folate levels due to malabsorption.

In the case of central nervous system (CNS) related Whipple's, a stereotactic brain biopsy is preferred. Endocardial biopsies are advised for cardiac involvement. Skeletal association may show evidence of changes similar to rheumatoid arthritis/ankylosing spondylitis.

Polymerase chain reaction (PCR) testing for *T whipplei* is currently the most specific diagnostic tool of choice.

Management

The management of choice relies on the use of trimethoprim sulfamethoxazole (TMX) long term (up to two years) in addition to benzylpenicillin. Folate replacement is advised due to malabsorption secondary to TMX. If there is associated CNS involvement, recommendations for the use of ceftriaxone and streptomycin exist. Response to treatment in general is seen following symptomatic improvement and repeated PCR testing.

Tropical Sprue

Aetiopathogenesis

It is unclear currently the precise cause of tropical sprue. Evidence suggests its prevalence in the tropics is due to bacterial infection and overgrowth leading to malabsorption in addition to altered bowel motility being seen. Bacteria such as *E coli* and *Enterobacter* have been noted.

Symptoms

- Symptoms secondary to malabsorption such as diarrhoea and weight loss
- Fever

Signs

- Weight loss
- Hypovolaemia

Differentials

- Coeliac disease
- Whipple's disease
- Bacterial overgrowth
- Intestinal lymphoma

Investigations

Blood investigations demonstrate evidence of anaemia with reduced folate and B12 levels. Electrolyte disturbance is common secondary to malabsorption. Patients may also demonstrate evidence of elevated faecal fat and reduced D-xylose excretion. Imaging analysis through the use of barium can often indicate the presence of thickened mucosal folds. Jejunal biopsy sampling as an invasive test may highlight the presence of villous atrophy and crypt formation.

Management

Management of tropical sprue relies on the replacement of fluid, electrolytes and nutrients with antibiotic use in the form of tetracycline.

Inflammatory
Bowel Disease (IBD)

Aetiopathogenesis

IBD has a significant genetic association comprising CARD15 (NOD2) on chromosome 16, OCTN1 and OCTN2 to name but a few. The HLA haplotype DRB1* 0103 has been linked with both ulcerative colitis (UC) and Crohn's disease. Studies have also shown that genetic mutations in the IL23 R gene may prove protective against Crohn's. Environmental factors are also important and studies have shown that breastfeeding is protective. An increased risk of IBD has been linked to excess consumption of carbohydrates and polyunsaturated fats. Lower levels of hygiene have been linked with a reduced risk of IBD as a result of a more effective immune-based response. Smoking has been linked with a reduction in UC and worsening Crohn's. Infective elements such as *Mycobacterium avium* may be associated with IBD.

Pathogenesis wise, antigens enter the underlying mucosa due to increased leakage within the epithelial barrier. This results in production of Th1 (Crohn's), Th17 and Th2 (UC) cells as well as NK cells. These cells release pro-inflammatory cytokines which stimulate macrophages to produce TNF alpha and IL1 and IL6. The end result is significant inflammatory damage. Pain and motility dysfunction are thought to be related to substance P and histamine to name but a few.

Symptoms
- Abdominal pain (typically right-sided in Crohn's)
- Perianal pain (typically seen in Crohn's due to fistulas and abscesses)
- Diarrhoea/constipation
- Mucus/blood PR (more typical in UC)
- Weight loss (more common in Crohn's due to malabsorption)
- Fever secondary to a flare

Signs
- Abdominal mass (typical in Crohn's)
- Perianal complications e.g. fissures, rectal prolapse, abscess (typical in Crohn's)
- Growth retardation (typical in younger patients)
- Fever
- Haemodynamic instability in the acute phase
- Extraintestinal manifestations such as iritis, episcleritis, evidence of arthropathy, dermatological disease (erythema nodosum, pyoderma gangrenosum, aphthous ulceration)

Differentials
- Coeliac disease
- Gastroenteritis
- IBS
- Diverticular disease

Investigations
Investigations of choice in the first instance include a FBC, U and E's, LFTs, CRP, as well as serum ferritin, B12 and folate (to determine classification of anaemia). Stools should be screened for calprotectin which helps to detect colonic inflammation as well as for MC and S and *C Difficile*. Screening for cytomegalovirus should be considered in severe or refractory disease states. Other useful tests comprise serology, namely

perinuclear anti-neutrophil cytoplasmic antibodies (pANCA) seen in UC and anti–saccharomyces cerevisiae antibodies (ASCA) in Crohn's. Imaging relies on an abdominal X-ray (AXR) initially to exclude toxic megacolon. Colonoscopy is the gold standard invasive test allowing for acquisition of biopsy samples. It is important to note, however, that in the acute phase the risk of perforation is high and therefore a flexible sigmoidoscopy may be the initial step. Barium studies allow for assessment of colonic abnormalities when endoscopy is limited or contraindicated. Additional imaging is usually in the form of MRI/CT enabling assessment of strictures, abscesses or fistulae as well as peri-anal disease.

Management

With reference to the British Society of Gastroenterology, active Crohn's disease relies on the use of prednisolone in the first instance. Failure to respond warrants the use of anti-tumour necrosis factor therapy such as infliximab or adalimumab. Infliximab is of particular benefit to patients with fistulating Crohn's. Contraindications include congestive cardiac failure and demyelinating disease. To help induce and maintain remission in less severe cases, alternative agents are also of benefit and include azathioprine, 6 Mercaptopurine and methotrexate.

Perianal Crohn's disease relies on the use of metronidazole or ciprofloxacin. Surgical interventional may also prove worthwhile.

Surgery for Crohn's disease in general is indicated in cases of failure to improve with medical therapy in addition to complications such as fibrosis and stenosis.

With regard to active ulcerative colitis, mesalazine is the initial drug of choice. This is followed by prednisolone if improvement fails to occur. In severe cases (patients with > 6 bloody stools/day and signs of systemic toxicity i.e. HR > 90/min, T > 37.8 °C, Hb < 10.5 g/dl or ESR > 30 mm/h), intravenous steroids are a requirement, in addition to appropriate fluid resuscitation and subcutaneous heparin in order to reduce the risk of thromboembolism. If after day 3 patients remain symptomatic, it is advisable to commence ciclosporin and infliximab, or proceed for urgent surgical intervention. In case of toxic megacolon (diameter > 5.5 cm), surgery is paramount. Maintenance of remission is typically with aminosalicylates, azathioprine or mercaptopurine.

In all cases, it is important to pay particular attention to nutritional deficits. In cases of short bowel syndrome or perioperatively, patients may require total parenteral nutrition (TPN).

Drug-related side effects

Due to the complexity of medical management, it is important to be aware of drug-related side effects:

Sulfasalazine — abdominal pain, diarrhoea, Stevens Johnson syndrome, pancreatitis, agranulocytosis

Mesalazine — diarrhoea, rash, renal failure

Steroids — moon face, oedema, sleep disturbance, glucose intolerance, osteoporosis, myopathy, osteonecrosis of the femoral head, adrenal insufficiency during withdrawal

Thiopurines — flu-like symptoms, leucopenia, liver failure, pancreatitis

Methotrexate — GI side effects e.g. diarrhoea, nausea, vomiting, liver failure, pneumonitis. Co-treatment with folic acid is advised

Ciclosporin — tremor, paraesthesia, liver dysfunction, gingival hyperplasia, hirsutism, renal failure, neurotoxicity, seizures (increased in patients with low serum cholesterol and magnesium)

Infliximab — infusion reactions, congestive cardiac failure, risk of overwhelming sepsis and malignancy

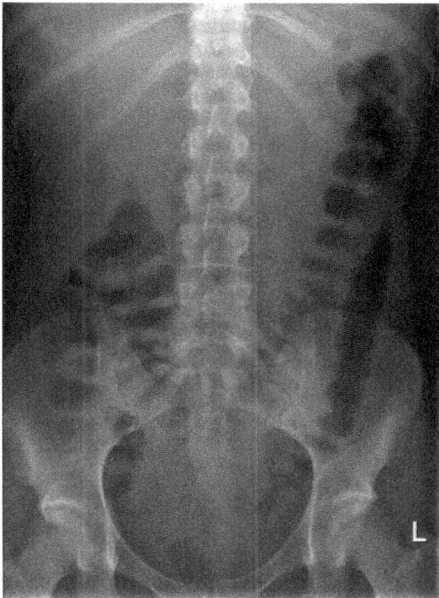

Fig. 4.   An abdominal X-ray demonstrating thickening of the descending and sigmoid colon in keeping with active colitis

Intestinal Ischaemia

Aetiopathogenesis

Cases of acute mesenteric ischaemia are typically due to arterial occlusion, with emboli to the superior mesenteric artery secondary to mural thrombi from cardiac hypokinesia or atrial fibrillation, cardiac valvular lesions or cholesterol embolization. Thrombosis is another cause for arterial occlusion, in addition to a dissecting aortic aneurysm, vasculitis or trauma. Non-occlusive mesenteric ischaemia occurs secondary to hypotension, cardiac failure or sepsis. Venous occlusion is evident and can occur secondary to protein C/S, antithrombin III or factor V Leiden deficiency, antiphospholipid syndrome or paroxysmal nocturnal haemoglobinuria. Additional causes include pancreatitis, IBD, cirrhosis or trauma.

Ischaemic colitis generally occurs due to inferior mesenteric artery thrombosis, mesenteric artery emboli or cholesterol emboli. Additional causes include shock, drugs such as antihypertensives, cocaine, methamphetamine, oestrogens or pseudoephedrine, coagulation disorders, vasculitis or cardiac/lower GI surgery.

Symptoms
- Abdominal pain (note in chronic mesenteric ischaemia this usually occurs post-prandially)
- Fever
- Diarrhoea
- Nausea
- Bleeding PR

Signs

- Abdominal tenderness/guarding
- Hypotension
- Tachycardia
- Melaena
- Signs of underlying cause e.g. atrial fibrillation

Differentials

- Abdominal abscess
- Abdominal aortic aneurysm
- Aortic dissection
- Biliary obstruction
- Colonic obstruction
- Diverticulitis
- Pancreatitis
- Pyelonephritis

Investigations

One of the primary blood investigations of choice is an arterial blood gas which will demonstrate evidence of a metabolic acidosis secondary to a rise in lactate. Additional investigations include a coagulation screen and FBC.

Imaging is important and should include a CT/MRI angiography which can help to demonstrate bowel wall thickening, submucosal oedema as well as vascular defects. It is important to note that even though an AXR is often requested in the first instance, they are often non-diagnostic and hence more advanced imaging is needed.

Management

Management is classically surgical with resection of infarcted bowel and embolectomy. There is merit for the use of an intra-arterial thrombolytic agent infusion such as streptokinase or tissue plasminogen activator in the acute setting. In non-occlusive cases, the vasodilator papaverine is worthwhile. For patients with a hypercoagulable state, treatment with heparin followed by long-term warfarin is needed.

Lower GI Bleeding

Aetiopathogenesis

The major causes of a lower GI bleed are detailed in Table 7.

Table 7: Major causes of colonic bleeding

Diverticular disease
Vascular malformations (angiodysplasia)
Ischaemic colitis
Haemorrhoids
Inflammatory bowel disease (e.g. ulcerative colitis, Crohn's disease)
Neoplasia (carcinoma or polyps)
Radiation enteropathy

Symptoms

- Bleeding PR, typically bright red if left-sided and painless if elderly with diverticular disease or angiodysplasia
- Abdominal pain particularly with ischaemic colitis
- Altered bowel habit in cases of colon cancer or IBD
- Mucus PR
- Weight loss

Signs

- Haemodynamic instability

Differentials

- Diverticular disease
- Ischaemic colitis
- Lower GI malignancy

Investigations

A colonoscopy is the gold standard investigation of choice. Blood investigations are much the same as that of an upper GI bleed. In addition to a colonoscopy, imaging in the form of a CT scan may prove beneficial in cases of suspected intestinal ischaemia and diverticular disease. In cases of continued bleeding and colonoscopy failure, mesenteric angiography is the tool of choice.

Management

Patients presenting with a lower GI bleed should undergo a colonoscopy with consideration of angiography as per Scottish Intercollegiate Guidelines Network guidance. If colonoscopy fails to achieve haemostasis, angiographic embolization is a potential salvage measure as well as surgical intervention.

Table 8:   Acute lower gastrointestinal bleeding — initial assessment protocol

Consider for discharge or non-admission with outpatient follow-up if:

- age < 60 years, and;
- no evidence of haemodynamic compromise, and;
  no evidence of gross rectal bleeding, and;
- an obvious anorectal source of bleeding on rectal examination/ sigmoidoscopy.

Consider for admission if:

- age ≥ 60 years, or;
- haemodynamic disturbance, or;
- evidence of gross rectal bleeding, or;
- taking aspirin or an NSAID, or;
- significant comorbidity.

Colorectal Cancer (CRC)

Aetiopathogenesis

Literature commonly cites the adenoma carcinoma sequence in the aetiopathogenesis of CRC. Adenomatous polyposis coli (APC) gene mutations are an initiating factor with subsequent KRAS oncogene activation and inactivation of TP53. Another factor of interest is the high level microsatellite instability (MS1-H) phenotype due to MLH 1 gene promoter methylation. Lynch syndrome demonstrates that evidence of MS1-H and familial adenomatous polyposis (FAP) is associated with the adenoma carcinoma sequence.

In terms of risk factors for disease causation, individuals with a history of IBD and diabetes are at increased risk. Smoking and alcohol intake are contributing factors in addition to an intake of red meat and lowered quantities of fibre/fruit and vegetables.

Symptoms

- Rectal bleeding
- Abdominal pain
- Bowel habit change
- It is important to note that right-sided lesions are associated with bleeding and predominantly diarrhoea with left-sided pathology linked to risk of bowel obstruction.

Signs

- Abdominal tenderness
- Bleeding PR

- Palpable abdominal mass
- Ascites
- Intestinal obstruction

Differentials

- IBD
- Diverticular disease
- Ischaemic bowel

Investigations

The investigation of choice includes a colonoscopy, which allows for a histological diagnosis. Patients with major comorbidities may undergo a flexible sigmoidoscopy and barium enema. Alternatives include a CT colonography. Staging is important and relies on CT of the chest, abdomen and pelvis. MRI or endorectal ultrasound is best suited for those with suspected rectal cancer. Of course patients must undergo blood investigations, comprising a FBC (to exclude anaemia), U and E's, LFTs (to exclude metastatic involvement) and serum CEA. The latter is typically taken preoperatively for prognostic purposes.

Table 9:   Risk of recurrence of rectal tumours as per MRI assessment

High	• A threatened (< 1 mm) or breached resection margin *or* • Low tumours encroaching onto the inter-sphincteric plane *or* with levator involvement
Moderate	• Any cT3b or greater, in which the potential surgical margin is not threatened *or* • Any suspicious lymph node not threatening the surgical resection margin *or* • The presence of extramural vascular invasion*
Low	• cT1 or cT2 or cT3a *and* • No lymph node involvement

*This feature is also associated with high risk of systemic recurrence.

Management

It is advisable to offer short-course preoperative radiotherapy, then immediate surgery for those with moderate-risk operable rectal cancer. For those that are bordering between moderate and high risk, consider preoperative chemoradiotherapy. This should also be considered for those with high-risk operable rectal cancer.

Patients presenting with obstructive-type symptoms require a colonic stent in the first instance.

In all cases of surgical intervention, patients should be assessed for the benefits of laparoscopic versus open resection.

Adjuvant chemotherapy is required in cases of high-risk stage II and stage III rectal cancer. Such treatment is also required in stage II patients post-surgery. Adjuvant chemotherapy for stage III cancer comprises capecitabine and oxaliplatin in combination with 5-Fluorouracil and folinic acid.

Metastatic disease relies on appropriate imaging through CT/MRI. Chemotherapy is the typical form of treatment in such cases and comprises oxaliplatin and irinotecan in combination with fluoropyrimidines. Examples of treatment include FOLFOX, FOLFIRI or XELOX. Raltitrexed should be instigated in those patients who are intolerant to 5-FU and folinic acid. An alternative option is also capecitabine or tegafur with uracil. It is important to note that the management of colorectal cancer requires multidisciplinary input and patients require surveillance colonoscopy one year after initial treatment and then five yearly if the primary investigation is normal.

Peutz Jeghers Syndrome (PJS)

Aetiopathogenesis

PJS is an autosomal dominant genetic condition associated with a STK11 mutation, a tumour suppressor gene. The primary role of STK11 is the regulation of cellular proliferation via G1 cell cycle arrest.

Symptoms

- Abdominal pain which is colicky in nature
- Bleeding PR
- Menstrual disturbance

Signs

- Mucocutaneous pigmentation
- Rectal mass
- Gynaecomastia
- Testicular mass

Differentials

- IBD
- Colonic malignancy
- Anal fissure
- Intussusception
- Rectal prolapse

Investigations

Blood investigations are an initial investigation of choice to help exclude the presence of anaemia courtesy of iron deficiency and potential liver metastases. An upper and lower GI endoscopy is essential in determining a diagnosis as well as consideration of video capsule endoscopy. Due to its multi-systemic association, evidence encourages genitalia assessment through ultrasound and cervical smear as well as breast assessment through MRI.

Management

Endoscopic polypectomy is advised to reduce cancer risk. Follow-up of all patients is essential and is detailed below:

General
- Annual FBC and LFT's
- Annual clinical examination

Genital tract
- Annual examination and testicular examination from birth until 12 years
- Testicular ultrasound if abnormalities detected at examination
- Cervical smear with liquid-based cytology (LBC) three-yearly from age 25 years

Gastrointestinal
- Baseline oesophago gastro duodenoscopy (OGD)/colonoscopy age 8
  — Polyps detected, continue three-yearly until 50 years
  — No polyps detected, repeat age 18 years, then three-yearly until 50 years
- Colonoscopy 1–2-yearly after age 50 years
- Video capsule endoscopy (VCE) three-yearly from age 8 years

Breast
- Monthly self-examination from age 18 years
- Annual breast MRI from age 25–50, thereafter annual mammography.

Familial Adenomatous Polyposis (FAP)

Aetiopathogenesis

FAP is an autosomal dominant genetic disorder associated with mutations of the adenomatous polyposis coli (APC) tumour suppressor gene localised to chromosome 5q. The primary function of APC is the promotion of apoptosis; however, subsequent mutations lead to mucosal hyperproliferation throughout the GI tract.

Symptoms

Symptoms are typically non-specific and may include:

- Abdominal pain
- Bleeding PR
- Diarrhoea

Signs

- Congenital hypertrophy of the retinal pigment epithelium which appears as pigmented lesions
- Osteomas indicative of Gardner's syndrome, seen commonly on the mandible. Dental abnormalities such as missing teeth, supernumerary or impacted teeth
- Epidermoid cysts located on the face, scalp or limbs
- Desmoid tumours
- Abdominal mass significant of small bowel or hepatobiliary malignancy

- Thyroid mass significant of malignancy
- CNS disturbance secondary to malignancy such as a glioblastoma/medulloblastoma

Differentials

- Peutz-Jeghers syndrome
- IBD
- Colonic malignancy

Investigations

An upper and lower GI endoscopy is helpful in determining the presence of polyps/malignancy. Imaging should also be undertaken in the form of an abdominal ultrasound/CT. In view of possible thyroid malignancy an ultrasound is also required. CNS disturbance should be investigated with a CT/MRI head scan to exclude malignancy. Dental abnormalities require appropriate X-ray imaging.

Management

Surgical intervention is essential in terms of polyp and tumour resection. For duodenal pathology, late-stage disease requires a duodenectomy. Sulindac in association with tamoxifen is beneficial for the treatment of desmoid lesions. Chemotherapy and radiotherapy are also useful in this regard.

It is important to note that follow-up of such patients is essential, and focusing on colorectal surveillance as the primary example, research suggests a 1–2 yearly sigmoidoscopy for patients with classical FAP.

TOPIC

Hereditary Non-Polyposis Colorectal Cancer (HNPCC)

Aetiopathogenesis

HNPCC occurs secondary to mutations in DNA mismatch repair genes. Such genes are responsible for correction of mismatches during DNA replication. Therefore a mutation promotes the formation of DNA damage and subsequent tumour formation within the GI tract and beyond. Common mismatch repair genes involved include MSH2, MLH1 and MSH6.

Symptoms
- Altered bowel habit: constipation/diarrhoea
- Bleeding PR
- Abdominal pain
- Weight loss
- Urinary symptoms
- Vaginal bleeding
- Dyspareunia

Signs
- Abdominal tenderness
- Cachexia
- Bleeding PR
- Bloody vaginal discharge

Differentials

- IBD
- Colorectal cancer
- PJS
- FAP

The Amsterdam criteria is utilised to aid in the diagnosis of HNPCC and comprises the following:

- Three or more family members with HNPCC-related malignancy
- Two successive affected generations
- One or more HNPCC-related malignancy diagnosed before the age of 50

Investigations

Patients suspected of the disease should undergo colonoscopy and immunohistochemistry/microsatellite instability testing for HNPCC. In view of extra colonic involvement, patients require an endometrial ultrasound, urine cytology analysis and an upper GI endoscopy.

Management

The use of aspirin has been shown to reduce the incidence of colorectal cancer occurrence. Intervention in the form of colonic and endometrial cancer resection is advised. A prophylactic hysterectomy is also beneficial. Follow-up of patients requires a three-yearly colonoscopy, with a 1–2-yearly colonoscopy for mutation carriers. Endometrial, urinary tract and upper GI screening should take place 1–2-yearly.

Diverticular Disease

Aetiopathogenesis

Research suggests that a diet low in fibre and high in red meat is one of the principle causes of diverticular disease. Additional associated risk factors exist and include smoking, NSAIDs and paracetamol use. The bowel undergoes several changes of non-compliance including increased muscularity and enhanced contractions, increased elastin deposition, and disturbed collagen composition. This leads to a rise in intra-colonic pressure and segmentation. The end result is herniation of portions of the colonic mucosa and submucosa at areas of weakness, typically caused by the vasa recta vasculature. Common sites of occurrence include the sigmoid colon due to its smaller diameter. Diverticulitis occurs following perforation of a diverticulum which is associated with worsening inflammation, abscess formation and peritonitis. Bleeding is seen secondary to rupture of colonic vasculature. The condition therefore comprises a spectrum of diverticula formation through to diverticulitis, and bleeding.

Symptoms

- Left lower abdominal pain, cramp-like in nature
- Altered bowel habit with constipation/diarrhoea and bleeding PR
- Nausea and vomiting
- Fever

Signs

- Abdominal tenderness with rebound and guarding
- Abdominal mass
- Bleeding PR

Differentials

- Appendicitis
- Cholecystitis
- Intestinal obstruction
- Peptic ulcer disease
- IBD/IBS
- Renal stones
- Pancreatitis
- Urinary tract infection

Investigations

Imaging investigations are essential and include an abdominal and chest X-ray. The former helps to determine the presence of obstruction/dilatation whereas the latter can guide to the existence of a pneumoperitoneum. An abdominal CT scan is the gold standard imaging tool, however, and helps to confirm the presence of diverticula, bowel wall thickening and abscess formation as well as colonic obstruction/fistula formation. Blood investigations are non-diagnostic but a full blood count should be performed to exclude infection as well as a renal screen to exclude evidence of electrolyte disturbance secondary to diarrhoea and vomiting.

Management

Patients with acute diverticulitis require the use of a low residue diet, in addition to antibiotics such as amoxicillin, sulfamethoxazole-trimethoprim, or a quinolone and metronidazole. In more severe cases, patients should receive adequate analgesia as well as fluid replacement. Surgical intervention is required in cases of perforation, obstruction, abscess and fistula formation.

Small and Large Bowel Obstruction (SBO/LBO)

Aetiopathogenesis

SBO is typically seen following surgery secondary to the presence of adhesions. Additional causes for the condition include the existence of a hernia, tumour or volvulus.

LBO is classically due to malignancy, strictures secondary to diverticular disease or ischaemia and volvulus.

In both cases, the existence of obstruction leads to bowel dilatation, increased pressure build-up and compression of the lymphatic system. The end result is the formation of oedema with third spacing of fluids and electrolytes within the bowel. Bacteria also tend to proliferate in close proximity to the obstruction in question.

Symptoms

In both cases:

- Abdominal pain which is cramp-like in nature
- Diarrhoea/Constipation/Flatus imbalance
- Nausea
- Vomiting

Signs

- Fever
- Tachycardia
- Abdominal distension and tenderness
- Hyperactive/diminished bowel sounds

- Rectal examination demonstrative of blood suggesting malignancy or strangulation, or a mass implying malignancy or impacted stool
- Inguinal or femoral hernias

Differentials

- Constipation
- IBD
- Diverticular disease
- Appendicitis

Investigations

Patients with SBO/LBO should undergo blood investigations to assess for electrolyte disturbance and an elevated urea and creatinine. A FBC will aid in determining the presence of infection, in addition to a lactate to exclude ischaemia/perforation. Imaging in the form of an abdominal X-ray will help to confirm the presence of dilated bowel loops and an air fluid level. More advanced imaging includes a CT/MRI scan to determine the presence of masses, abscesses or evidence of ischaemia/strangulation. The use of a water-soluble contrast enema has been shown to provide imaging and therapeutic advantage in both SBO and LBO.

Management

SBO requires fluid replacement and decompression in the first instance along with antibiotics, anti-emetics and analgesia. Surgical intervention is often required in cases of strangulation.

LBO follows similar management to SBO with a need for fluid resuscitation, decompression via a nasogastric (NG) tube and antibiotics. Surgical treatment is instigated in cases which are more acute in presentation such as closed loop obstruction and ischaemia.

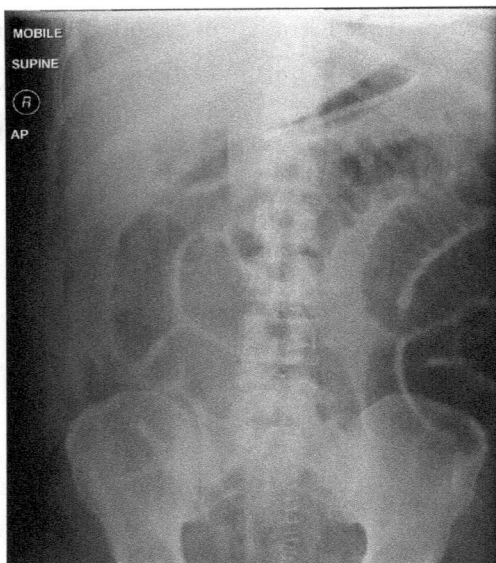

Fig. 5.   Abdominal X-ray demonstrating small bowel obstruction

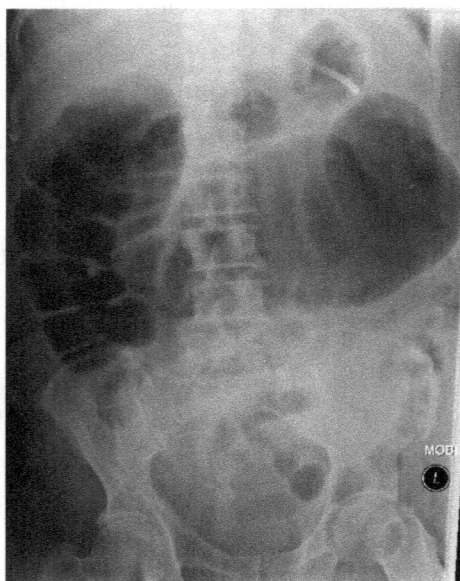

Fig. 6.   Abdominal X-ray demonstrating large bowel obstruction

Carcinoid Syndrome

Aetiopathogenesis

Carcinoid syndrome occurs secondary to the release of kinins and sero-tonin from tumours arising from neuroendocrine cells. These cells are typically found deep within the mucosa.

Symptoms

- Flushing affecting the face and upper trunk
- Diarrhoea
- Wheezing secondary to broncho pulmonary carcinoid
- Abdominal pain
- Chest pain

Signs

- Tachycardia
- Hypertension or hypotension
- Confusion
- Valvular heart disease

Differentials

- Anaphylaxis
- Angioedema
- Tumour lysis syndrome

Investigations

Patients should undergo urinary measurement of 5 hydroxyindoleacetic acid (5 HIAA) which is produced following the metabolism of serotonin. An abdominal ultrasound scan aids in the detection of potential metastases. Additional tests of choice may include measurement of serum chromogranin A as well as octreotide scanning for staging purposes.

Management

Management relies on the use of somatostatin analogues such as octreotide and lanreotide as well as interferon alpha. Curative treatment is surgical in nature, particularly in early-stage disease.

Neuroendocrine Tumours (NETs)

Aetiopathogenesis

NETs arise from neuroendocrine cells which derive from local multi-potent gastrointestinal stem cells courtesy of an array of transcription factors. Most tumours develop sporadically but a genetic association is noted, case in point, MEN1 syndrome. However the precise molecular aspects of such tumours are poorly understood with limited information from animal models.

Symptoms and Signs

Symptoms are tumour type-dependent:

- VIPoma — significant watery diarrhoea, abdominal cramps
- Insulinoma — sweats, dizziness, weakness, which improve with eating
- Gastrinoma — diarrhoea and abdominal pain, secondary to peptic ulceration (Zollinger Ellison syndrome)
- Glucagonoma — weight loss, diarrhoea, increasing thirst and urinary frequency secondary to diabetes, necrolytic migratory erythema, stomatitis
- Somatostatinoma — weight loss, diarrhoea, steatorrhoea, increasing thirst and urinary frequency secondary to diabetes, abdominal pain secondary to gallstones (cholecystokinin inhibition by somatostatin)

Note that carcinoid syndrome was discussed previously.

Differentials

Differentials in this regard comprise the above listed NETs subtypes.

Investigations

Blood investigations of choice include chromogranin A and urinary 5 HIAA as well as pancreatic polypeptide, which are likely to be raised. Depending on the suspected tumour type, further serum tests should be requested e.g. gastrin, somatostatin, glucagon, VIP and insulin. Urea and electrolytes are of value in the case of a VIPoma in view of diarrhoea leading to severe hypokalaemia. Imaging is essential and can include a CT/MRI and somatostatin receptor scintigraphy, in addition to PET scanning. Additional imaging of choice should include an endoscopic ultrasound. Histology of course determines the final diagnosis.

Management

Management relies on surgical intervention for cases which are deemed resectable. For non-surgical patients, treatment relies on somatostatin analogues, biotherapy, radionuclide therapy, ablation and chemotherapy. For patients with advanced disease, namely inoperable or metastatic in nature, therapies such as sunitinib (tyrosine kinase inhibitor of vascular endothelial and platelet-derived growth factor) or everolimus (protein kinase inhibitor of mTOR) should be employed. In metastatic cases, small volume tumours can benefit from ablation.

Acute Appendicitis

Aetiopathogenesis

The primary factor responsible for acute appendicitis is secondary to obstruction of the appendiceal lumen. This can occur as a result of lymphoid hyperplasia as seen in IBD, infection, malignancy or the presence of faecoliths. Over time such obstruction leads to a rise in intraluminal pressure and further bacterial colonisation and inflammation.

Symptoms

- Abdominal pain which is colicky and central initially with radiation to the right iliac fossa
- Loss of appetite
- Nausea and vomiting
- Constipation

Signs

- Fever
- Tachycardia
- Abdominal tenderness with rebound. Site of maximal tenderness localised to McBurney's point (two thirds of the way along a line drawn from the umbilicus to the anterior superior iliac spine). Rovsing's sign is also observed where palpation of the left iliac fossa causes pain in the right.

Differentials

- Intestinal obstruction
- Peptic ulcer

- Intussusception
- Pancreatitis
- Renal colic
- Ectopic pregnancy
- Pelvic inflammatory disease
- Gastroenteritis

Investigations

Investigations of choice include a FBC and CRP to exclude evidence of infection. In addition, patients should undergo a urinalysis and women of child-bearing age should have a pregnancy test. Imaging tools of choice include an ultrasound but more specifically a CT/MRI.

Management

Management relies on adequate fluid resuscitation, antibiotic use and surgical intervention. Laparoscopic surgery is typically preferred due to reduced complications and enhanced recovery time. Antibiotics used are of course dependent on local policy but classes of value include penicillin, cephalosporins or aminoglycosides.

Nutrition

For the purpose of this text, the following section has been included to highlight the evidence regarding enteral and parenteral nutrition:

Enteral nutrition is advised when oral intake is inadequate or not suitable, for example in those patients with dysphagia, in patients where the GI tract is functional. The process relies on feed being introduced into the stomach, duodenum or jejunum. If enteral forms of feed are not being tolerated due to delayed gastric emptying for example, a motility agent can be commenced. For patients on enteral nutrition, NG tube placement should be assessed via X-ray and pH testing. Gastrostomy/jejunostomy tubes should undergo assessment at the site of insertion to monitor position and exclude infection.

Parenteral nutrition should commence when oral or enteral intake is limited and/or the GI tract is non-functional in nature. A peripheral venous catheter is used in short-term cases with a tunnelled subclavian line preferred for long-term use. The site of catheter insertion should be assessed for the presence of infection.

Enteral nutrition is usually ceased when oral intake is sufficient, and parenteral when enteral or oral intake is adequate.

All patients on nutritional support require appropriate blood investigations, including for renal and liver function, serum glucose, magnesium, phosphate, calcium, vitamin D, albumin, zinc, copper, selenium and manganese, a FBC, CRP, mean corpuscular volume (MCV) and iron/ferritin/folate/B12 levels.

Refeeding Syndrome

Aetiopathogenesis

Refeeding Syndrome (RS) is seen typically following rapid refeeding whether enteral or parenteral following the occurrence of nutritional deficit. During starvation, the body utilises fat and protein as an energy source. During the refeeding process, carbohydrate loading occurs and the rise in blood glucose results in increased insulin and decreased glucagon secretion resulting in glycogen, fat and protein synthesis. This requires minerals such as phosphate and magnesium as well as thiamine. The presence of insulin results in potassium absorption into the cells courtesy of the sodium potassium ATPase symporter. Magnesium and phosphate are also transported into the cells. The clinical features of refeeding syndrome therefore occur due to the significant electrolyte deficit.

Symptoms

Symptoms are primarily related to electrolyte disturbance. In a broad sense, patients may experience:

- Chest pain
- Shortness of breath
- Muscular weakness
- Fatigue
- Confusion
- Fits

Signs

- Cardiac arrhythmia
- Signs of cardiac failure
- Neurological disturbance

Differentials

- Hyperthyroidism
- IBS
- Intestinal malabsorption
- Protein-losing enteropathy

Investigations

All patients suspected of refeeding syndrome require regular blood investigations comprising a full electrolyte screen, paying particular attention to phosphate, magnesium, sodium and potassium. Serum glucose monitoring is also required.

Management

In view of the electrolyte disturbance, patients require intravenous replacement. This should be done in conjunction with appropriate nutritional specialists. It is important to identify those at high risk of refeeding syndrome in the first instance. These include patients with a BMI < 18 kg/m^2, unintentional weight loss > 10–15%, minimal nutritional intake prior to refeeding, and a history of alcohol, insulin, chemotherapy or diuretic use.

Jaundice

Aetiopathogenesis

Jaundice is classified as pre-hepatic, hepatic or post-hepatic, and tends to occur with a bilirubin concentration > 40 micromol/l. Pre-hepatic jaundice is associated with excess unconjugated bilirubin which is insoluble and so does not appear in the urine. The primary underlying cause is haemolysis and it is commonly linked to sickle cell disease and thalassaemia.

Hepatic causes of jaundice comprise viral hepatitis, alcoholic cirrhosis, primary biliary cirrhosis (PBC) and drugs such as analgesics. Post-hepatic jaundice is linked to the presence of biliary obstruction such as a stone or stricture of the biliary ductal system or pancreatic carcinoma. In post-hepatic jaundice, bilirubin is conjugated and hence appears in the urine leading to a darker appearance as well as paler stools. Hepatic jaundice is associated with a mixed bilirubin picture.

Symptoms
- Yellowing of skin/sclerae
- Abdominal pain
- Weight loss
- Pruritus

Signs
- Yellowing of skin/sclerae
- Brown urine (conjugated)

- Abdominal tenderness
- Gray coloured stools (conjugated)
- Hypotonia, deafness, oculomotor palsy (CN (Crigler Najjar) syndrome type 2)

Differentials

- Acute liver failure
- Alcoholic hepatitis
- Autoimmune hepatitis
- Biliary obstruction
- Cholangiocarcinoma
- Cholecystitis
- Cirrhosis
- Haemochromatosis
- Pancreatitis
- Pancreatic cancer
- Iron deficiency anaemia
- Pernicious anaemia
- Lead toxicity

Investigations

Investigations of choice include a FBC, LFTs, coagulation, hepatitis and autoimmune screen, iron and copper studies, and screens for alcohol, paracetamol and alpha 1 anti-trypsin levels. Procedural investigations include an abdominal ultrasound scan, an abdominal CT, a liver biopsy, an endoscopic retrograde cholangio pancreatogram (ERCP)/and a percutaneous transhepatic cholangiogram (PTC).

Management

Jaundice management relies on determining the status of hyperbilirubinaemia as either conjugated or unconjugated. Treatment of conjugated hyperbilirubinaemia relies on focusing on the underlying cause. With regard to unconjugated hyperbilirubinaemia, treatment is as follows:

- Gilbert's syndrome — symptomatic relief
- CN syndrome type 1 — plasma exchange and phototherapy due to risk of encephalopathy. Liver transplantation is, however, the definitive treatment of choice.
- CN syndrome type 2 — Phenobarbital
- Neonatal jaundice — phototherapy

Ascites

Aetiopathogenesis

Vasodilation is the underlying trigger for the development of ascites. Evidence suggests that increased hepatic resistance to portal flow secondary to cirrhosis leads to the development of portal hypertension, collateral vein formation and shunting of blood to the systemic circulation. The production of nitric oxide leads to splanchnic arterial vasodilation and eventually sodium and fluid retention. The accumulation of fluid within the abdominal cavity is linked to altered intestinal capillary pressure and permeability.

Symptoms

- Abdominal swelling

Signs

- Chronic liver disease
- Hepatomegaly
- Elevated JVP
- Anasarca

Differentials

- Acute liver failure
- Alcoholic hepatitis
- Cardiomyopathy
- Cirrhosis
- Viral hepatitis

- Hepatocellular cancer
- Hepatorenal syndrome
- Nephrotic syndrome
- Primary biliary cirrhosis
- Portal hypertension

Investigations

Investigating ascites relies on determining the serum ascites-albumin gradient (SA-AG). See Table 10.

Table 10:   Serum ascites-albumin gradient (SA-AG)

SA-AG ≥ 11g/l	SA-AG < 11g/l
Cirrhosis	Malignancy
Cardiac failure	Pancreatitis
Nephrotic syndrome	Tuberculosis

It is advised that ascitic amylase should be measured when one suspects pancreatic disease. In addition, ascitic fluid should be placed in blood culture bottles and sent for MC and S and neutrophil count analysis. Additional investigations of choice include an abdominal ultrasound scan.

Management

Treatment is governed by the serum sodium level as shown in Table 11.

Table 11: Treatment of ascites with serum sodium

Serum sodium 126–135 mmol/l, normal creatinine	Continue diuretics
Serum sodium 121–125 mmol/l, normal serum creatinine	Stop diuretic therapy
Serum sodium 121–125 mmol/l, serum creatinine elevated	Stop diuretics and volume expand
Serum sodium < 120 mmol/l	Stop diuretics. Volume expand with colloid/saline

First line treatment of ascites includes spironolactone. If this fails to provide benefit, then patients should be commenced on furosemide. Patients with large volume or refractory ascites require therapeutic paracentesis. Albumin is often given post-completion as a form of volume expansion. Individuals requiring frequent therapeutic paracentesis should undergo transjugular intrahepatic portosystemic shunting (TIPS). Patients with cirrhotic ascites should undergo liver transplantation.

Spontaneous bacterial peritonitis is worth a mention at this point. In patients with an ascitic fluid neutrophil count of > 250 cells/mm^3, antibiotic therapy is required. This comprises third-generation cephalosporins such as cefotaxime. Those with evidence of renal failure should be given albumin. Prophylaxis against spontaneous bacterial peritonitis (SBP) relies on norfloxacin or ciprofloxacin. And it goes without saying that those with SBP should be considered for liver transplantation.

Acute Liver Failure

Aetiopathogenesis

Acute liver failure can occur secondary to a multitude of factors. Examples include viral hepatitis, herpes simplex virus, varicella zoster virus, Epstein Barr virus, cytomegalovirus and parvovirus B19. Drug-related damage is common and includes paracetamol, NSAIDs, statins, anti-epileptics, anti-TB drugs and antibiotics such as amoxicillin and nitrofurantoin.

Symptoms

- Abdominal pain
- Confusion/tremor
- Abdominal distension
- Haematemesis/melaena in view of an upper GI bleed

Signs

- Stigmata of chronic liver disease
- Jaundice
- Abdominal tenderness
- Ascites
- Encephalopathy see Table 12
- Haemodynamic instability

Differentials

- Cirrhosis
- Autoimmune hepatitis

- Alcoholic hepatitis
- Sepsis

Table 12: West Haven criteria: signs/symptoms

❑ Changes in behavior with minimal change in level of consciousness +1

❑ Gross disorientation, drowsiness, possibly asterixis, inappropriate behavior +2

❑ Marked confusion, incoherent speech, sleeping most of the time but arousable to vocal stimuli +3

❑ Comatose, unresponsive to pain; decorticate or decerebrate posturing +4

Investigations

Initial investigations comprise a FBC (to exclude thrombocytopenia), U and E's (to exclude hepatorenal syndrome and hypophosphatemia), LFTs, coagulation profile, arterial pH (due to the risk of metabolic acidosis), screens for lactate, glucose (as hypoglycaemia is common), ammonia and paracetamol levels, toxicology screen, hepatitis serology, ceruloplasmin level, blood cultures and an autoimmune screen. A liver biopsy may be needed in cases of suspected autoimmune hepatitis but be mindful of concurrent coagulopathy. Imaging is worthwhile and can comprise a liver ultrasound with Doppler or CT to assess hepatic structure, the presence of ascites and vascular abnormalities.

Management

It is often advisable to liaise with intensive care for all patients admitted with acute liver failure. In cases of encephalopathy patients should be treated with lactulose in order to reduce ammonia levels. Sources of infection should be localised and treated accordingly. Such patients are often hyponatraemic and the use of hypertonic saline is of benefit. In case of coagulopathy, it is advisable to treat with vitamin K or fresh frozen plasma (FFP)/platelets in case of active bleeding. Cases of acute liver failure are accompanied by altered haemodynamics. Therefore, it is essential that fluid resuscitation/pressor support is instigated. Feeding is also paramount and should rely on enteral replacement where possible.

A requirement for liver transplantation is based on the King's College Criteria depicted in Table 13.

Table 13:   Potentially helpful indicators* of poor (transplant-free) prognosis in patients with acute liver failure

Aetiology
Idiosyncratic drug injury
Acute hepatitis B (and other non-hepatitis A viral infections)
Autoimmune hepatitis
Mushroom poisoning
Wilson disease
Budd-Chiari syndrome
Indeterminate cause
Coma grade on admission
III
IV
King's College Criteria:
Acetaminophen-induced acute liver failure:
Arterial pH < 7.3 (following adequate volume resuscitation) irrespective of coma grade OR
PT > 100 seconds (INR · 6.5) + serum creatinine > 300μmol/L (3.4 mg/dL) in patients in grade III/IV coma
Non-acetaminophen-induced acute liver failure:
PT >100 seconds irrespective of coma grade OR
Any three of the following, irrespective of coma grade:
— Drug toxicity, in determinate cause of acute liver failure
— Age < 10 years or > 40 years[‡]
— Jaundice to coma interval > 7 days[‡]
— PT > 50 seconds (INR ≥ 3.5)
— Serum bilirubin > 300 μmol/L (17.5 mg/dL)

*Please note: None of these factors with the exception of Wilson disease and possibly mushroom poisoning, are either necessary or sufficient to indicate the need for immediate liver transplantation.

[‡]These criteria, in particular, have not been found to be predictive of outcome in recent analyses.

Hepatorenal Syndrome (HRS)

Aetiopathogenesis

HRS is seen as a consequence of portal hypertension in cirrhosis. This leads to increased splanchnic production of vasodilators, namely nitric oxide, resulting in severe arterial underfilling, activation of the renin angiotensin system and impaired renal perfusion and glomerular filtration rate (GFR).

Symptoms

- Fatigue
- Malaise
- Reduced urine output

Signs

Stigmata of chronic liver disease as described previously

Differentials

- Acute tubular necrosis
- Glomerulonephritis

Investigations

Blood investigations of choice include a serum urea and creatinine, with Type 1 HRS being defined as a serum creatinine > 221 micromol/l in less than two weeks. Type 2 HRS demonstrates a serum creatinine on average of 178 micromol/l. In both cases glomerular filtration rate is reduced. Additional investigations of interest demonstrate a low urine volume < 500 ml/day, a low urine sodium, high urine osmolality, elevated urine protein and low serum sodium. Of course patients should undergo a FBC to exclude infection as well as a liver function screen. Imaging of choice comprises an abdominal ultrasound scan with Doppler flow for vascular assessment.

Management

Management of HRS is type-dependent. Type 1 patients are suitable candidates for liver transplantation as a high priority. Vasoconstrictors such as terlipressin should be commenced in addition to intravenous albumin. For those where vasoconstrictors have failed to provide benefit, transjugular intrahepatic portosystemic shunt should be undertaken. In case of renal complications such as pulmonary oedema, hypokalaemia, or metabolic acidosis, renal replacement should be commenced.

Patients with type 2 HRS should also be considered for liver transplantation. Diuretics should be instigated for ascites management and sodium restriction introduced. Repeated paracentesis in addition to intravenous albumin is required for the treatment of tense ascites. Fluid replacement should be restricted in the case of hyponatremia with the use of vasoconstrictors or TIPS prior to transplantation.

Alcoholic Liver Disease (ALD)

Aetiopathogenesis

The metabolism of alcohol relies on its breakdown to acetaldehyde and later to acetate. Alcohol aids in the translocation of lipopolysaccharide (LPS) from the small and large intestine to the portal vein and hence the liver. LPS within Kupffer cells binds to CD14, leading eventually to activation of cytokine genes; examples include TNF alpha, IL 8, MCP 1, platelet derived growth factor and TGF β, inducing inflammation. The end result is the activation of hepatic stellate cells leading to fibrosis.

It is also noted that the occurrence of lipid peroxidation secondary to alcohol metabolism associates with acetaldehyde, leading to the formation of neoantigens which induce an autoimmune-based response.

Symptoms

- Nausea
- Malaise
- Fever
- Abdominal pain
- Confusion
- Fits
- Haematemesis

Signs

- Haemodynamic instability
- Hepatomegaly
- Darkening of urine

- Splenomegaly
- Asterixis
- Oedema
- Ascites
- Jaundice
- Spider naevi

Differentials

- Viral hepatitis
- Chronic pancreatitis

Investigations

Recommended investigations comprise biochemistry and ultrasound platforms, in addition to a liver biopsy. However, the latter should not be instigated in cases of impaired coagulation. Studies have shown that an AST/ALT ratio >1 is universal in those with ALD. Such patients also require a full liver screen (see Acute Liver Failure for further information) as well as an infection screen comprising blood, ascites and urine culture in addition to U and E's to exclude hepatorenal syndrome. A FBC helps to exclude infection and existence of thrombocytosis/penia.

Management

Management in the first instance relies on prognostic scoring tools, primarily Maddrey's discriminant function and the Model for End-stage Liver Disease (MELD) score as exampled in Tables 14 and 15, respectively.

Table 14:   Maddrey's DF

PT	sec
PT control/Reference level	sec
Bilirubin	mg/dL

Table 15:   MELD score

Dialysis at least twice in the past week	❏ Yes ❏ NO
Creatinine	mg/dL
Bilirubin	mg/dL
INR	

Patients are then treated with either prednisolone or pentoxifylline (note if DF > 32). It is important to note that in cases of sepsis or GI bleeding, prednisolone should be avoided. N-acetylcysteine (NAC) may be useful in patients with severe alcoholic steatohepatitis on corticosteroid treatment.

In view of progression to alcoholic cirrhosis, patients must abstain from alcohol completely. Referral for liver transplantation requires a six month period of abstinence and is typically recommended in those with a Child-Pugh score of C and MELD score >15.

Hepatitis B

Aetiopathogenesis

Infected blood and semen are the primary methods of transmission. Sources of the former include injections, blood transfusion or dialysis. With regard to the latter, male-to-male intercourse as well as those who engage with multiple partners in an unprotected fashion are notable sources. The virus itself induces an innate immune response and is primarily a double stranded DNA virus. The persistent effects of the virus are maintained courtesy of cccDNA. Mutations of the virus are courtesy of single and double nucleotide changes. The end result of such mutations is the reduced formation of hepatitis B e-antigen (HBeAg) leading to HBeAg-negative chronic hepatitis B virus (HBV) infection. The phases of chronic infection are as follows:

- Immune tolerant: HBeAg-positive, elevated HBV DNA, typically normal aminotransferase
- HBeAg-positive chronic HBV infection: as above with subsequent aminotransferase dysfunction
- Inactive HBV carrier: HBeAg-negative, anti-HBe-positive, low levels of HBV DNA, normal aminotransferase
- HBeAg-negative: HBeAg-negative, HBV DNA moderately elevated, increased aminotransferase levels
- Resolved infection: HBsAg-negative, undetectable HBV DNA, normal aminotransferase levels, anti-HBc and anti-HBs

Symptoms

- Nausea
- Muscle weakness
- Fatigue
- Abdominal pain
- Joint discomfort

Signs

- Jaundice
- Hepatomegaly/splenomegaly
- Signs of chronic liver disease
- Pleural effusion
- Arrhythmia
- Neurological dysfunction e.g. Guillain-Barré syndrome/mononeuritis multiplex
- Maculopapular rash

Differentials

- Alcoholic hepatitis
- Autoimmune hepatitis
- Cholangitis
- Viral hepatitis
- Haemochromatosis
- Hepatocelluar carcinoma (HCC)

Investigations

Investigations of choice include screening for hepatitis B surface antigen (to determine the existence of acute hepatitis B), hepatitis B e-antigen (to determine degree of infectivity), HBV DNA level for the same reason, IgM antibody to hepatitis B core antigen (to determine the existence of acute hepatitis B), hepatitis C virus antibody, hepatitis D virus antibody, HIV antibody and IgG antibody to hepatitis A. Of course all patients should undergo a FBC, LFTs, clotting screen, alpha fetoprotein (AFP) scan and abdominal ultrasound scan. A transient elastography is required with subsequent liver biopsy in those with a score between 6 and 10 kPa.

Management

Chronic hepatitis B patients (either HBeAg-positive or HBeAg-negative) with compensated liver disease should be offered a 48-week course of peginterferon alfa 2a. Second-line treatment relies on tenofovir or entecavir. For pregnant or breastfeeding women, the drug of choice is tenofovir instigated typically in the third trimester. Patients on immunosuppressive therapy who are HBsAg-positive and have HBV DNA > 2000 IU/l should be given prophylaxis with entecavir or tenofovir for a minimum of six months. Individuals should be given lamivudine if their immunosuppressive therapy is expected to last less than six months.

Hepatitis C

Aetiopathogenesis

The literature cites two main primary modes of transmission of hepatitis C, which as is the case with hepatitis B, include contaminated blood and sexually related practices.

Research has shown that the existence of hepatitis C virus (HCV) helps to activate the innate immune system resulting in impaired toll-like receptor (TLR) signalling linked to HCV NS3/4A protease leading to chronic infection long term.

Symptoms

- Abdominal pain
- Pruritus
- Joint discomfort
- Weakness: sensory or muscular-related

Signs

- Signs of chronic liver disease
- Porphyria cutanea tarda
- Cryoglobulinaemia
- Lichen planus
- Purpura
- Keratoconjunctivitis sicca
- Necrotizing vasculitis

Differentials

- Autoimmune hepatitis

- Cholangitis
- Viral hepatitis

Investigations

In addition to the routine LFTs and coagulation screen, screening for anti-HCV is key in determining a diagnosis. Serum PCR testing is also recommended in patients suspected of HCV who are immune deficient. Additional testing comprises screening for antinuclear antibody (ANA), rheumatoid factor, anticardiolipin antibody, antithyroid antibody and anti-smooth muscle antibody to exclude autoimmune-based factors. Additional investigations of choice include a liver biopsy to determine the existence of fibrosis.

Management

Consensus recommendations for the treatment of Hepatitis C were published as below:

HCV genotype 1a-naïve patients should be treated with 12 weeks of interferon alpha 2a or 2b, with ribavirin and sofosbuvir, or 12 weeks of simeprevir and 24 weeks of pegylated interferon alpha 2a or 2b and ribavirin or faldaprevir for 12 weeks and pegylated interferon alpha 2a and ribavirin for 24 weeks.

HCV genotype 1b-naïve patients should be treated with either 12 weeks of interferon alpha 2a or 2b, with ribavirin and sofosbuvir, or treated with 12 weeks of simeprevir and 24 weeks of interferon alpha 2a or 2b and ribavirin or faldaprevir for 12 weeks and pegylated interferon alpha 2a and ribavirin for 24 weeks.

HCV genotype 1a or 1b treatment-experienced patients should be treated with either simeprevir for 12 weeks plus 24 or 48 weeks of interferon and ribavirin, especially if they relapsed on previous treatment or treated with 12 weeks of interferon alpha 2a or 2b, with ribavirin and sofosbuvir.

HCV genotype 1a or 1b with cirrhosis or severe fibrosis should be treated with 12 weeks of interferon alpha 2a or 2b, with ribavirin and sofosbuvir.

HCV genotype 2-naïve patients should be treated with 12 weeks of ribavirin and sofosbuvir.

HCV genotype 2 patients should be treated with 12 weeks of ribavirin and sofosbuvir.

HCV genotype 2 with cirrhosis or severe fibrosis could be treated with 12 weeks of ribavirin and sofosbuvir.

HCV genotype 3-naïve patients could be treated with either 12 weeks of pegylated interferon and ribavirin and sofosbuvir or treated with 24 weeks of pegylated interferon and ribavirin or 24 weeks of sofosbuvir and ribavirin.

HCV genotype 3 treatment-experienced patients could be offered 24 weeks of sofosbuvir and ribavirin or 12 weeks of pegylated interferon and ribavirin and sofosbuvir.

Patients with cirrhosis or severe fibrosis HCV genotype 3 could be offered 24 weeks of sofosbuvir and ribavirin or 12 weeks of sofosbuvir and ribavirin and interferon alpha, with similar efficacy.

HCV genotype 4 patients could be treated with 12 weeks of interferon alpha 2a or 2b, with ribavirin and sofosbuvir. Alternatively, they could be treated with simeprevir for 12 weeks plus 24 or 48 weeks of interferon and ribavirin.

HCV genotype 4, 5 or 6 treatment-experienced patients could be treated with either 12 weeks of interferon alpha 2a or 2b, with ribavirin and sofosbuvir or simeprevir with 24–48 weeks of interferon alpha 2a or 2b, with ribavirin.

HCV genotype 4, 5 or 6 with cirrhosis or severe fibrosis could be treated with 12 weeks of interferon alpha 2a or 2b, with ribavirin and sofosbuvir.

Side effects of interferon therapy include flu-like symptoms, myelosuppression and neuropsychiatric dysfunction. Ribavirin therapy is complicated by haemolysis. The pegylated form of interferon has been shown to be associated with an improvement in quality of life. Sofosbuvir has been linked to anaemia, fatigue, nausea and headaches. Simeprevir is associated with influenza-type symptoms and pruritus. Faldaprevir can lead to GI disturbance, rash and pruritus.

Hepatitis A, D and E

Aetiopathogenesis

Viral hepatitis A is an RNA virus transmitted via the faecal-oral route and sexually. Hepatitis D is also an RNA-based virus transmitted typically via blood, or sexually. Chronicity is notable in this case. This virus relies on the hepatitis B surface antigen in order to transmit its genome. Hepatitis E is transmitted via the faecal-oral route and is an RNA composite, as is the case with A and D. Progression to fulminant hepatic failure in pregnant women with hepatitis E has been observed. Fulminant liver failure in hepatitis A is, however, rare.

Symptoms

- Abdominal discomfort
- Jaundice
- Nausea
- Vomiting
- Muscle weakness
- Fatigue
- Headache
- Diarrhoea (pale in nature)
- Dark urine

Signs

- Hepatomegaly
- Splenomegaly

- Jaundice
- Lymphadenopathy
- Rash

Differentials

- Autoimmune hepatitis
- Alcoholic hepatitis
- Epstein Barr virus
- Cytomegalovirus
- Hepatitis B and C

Investigations

Blood investigations may demonstrate evidence of leucopenia, anaemia and thrombocytopenia. LFTs will demonstrate a rise in bilirubin and aminotransferase levels. A coagulation screen should of course be ordered. Hepatitis A patients demonstrate anti-hepatitis A IgM. Hepatitis D patients should undergo screening for hepatitis D antigen and RNA levels as well as anti-hepatitis D IgM. Hepatitis E patients should undergo testing for RNA levels as well as anti-hepatitis E IgM.

A liver ultrasound should be performed to assess for any other underlying pathology.

Management

Management of hepatitis A is generally conservative in nature with intravenous fluids and anti-emetics. Treatment of hepatitis D and E is also conservative in nature.

Non-Alcoholic Fatty Liver Disease (NAFLD)

Aetiopathogenesis

NAFLD is linked to obesity, type II diabetes and hyperlipidaemia. Additional factors that predispose to disease occurrence include protein malnutrition and total parenteral nutrition use, drugs such as steroids, oestrogen, amiodarone, tamoxifen and antiretrovirals.

Insulin resistance linked to inhibition of molecular factors such as Ras associated with diabetes, PC 1 and TNF alpha leads to the accumulation of fat within hepatocytes secondary to lipolysis. Increased uptake of fatty acids results in overload of mitochondrial β oxidation leading to further accumulation of fatty acids. Insulin resistance leads to glycolysis, further augmenting triglyceride deposition within hepatocytes by decreasing the production of apolipoprotein B 100. In addition, fatty acids function as a source of oxidative stress resulting in enhanced inflammation courtesy of cytokine production and cell apoptosis.

Research also demonstrates that fatty acid oxidation is regulated by peroxisome proliferator-activated receptor alpha (PPAR-alpha), which has been implicated in further hepatocyte damage.

Symptoms

- Fatigue
- Abdominal discomfort

Signs

- Abdominal tenderness
- Hepatomegaly

- Central adiposity
- Hypertension
- Acanthosis nigricans secondary to insulin resistance

Differentials

- Alcoholic hepatitis
- Cirrhosis
- Viral hepatitis

Investigations

Investigations of choice include a FBC and liver function screen to demonstrate evidence of elevated aminotransferase levels and absence of viral hepatitis. The gold standard diagnostic tool is a liver biopsy. Imaging in the form of an ultrasound and/or MRI is worthwhile.

Management

Management of NAFLD relies on addressing lifestyle factors in the first instance with weight reduction and control of serum glucose and lipid levels. Medication use in the form of metformin, gemfibrozil or vitamin E has been shown to be beneficial.

Bariatric surgical intervention in refractory cases is advised, aiding in the reduction of inflammation and fibrosis formation.

Cirrhosis

Aetiopathogenesis

Cirrhosis is the end result of chronic inflammation and hepatic stellate cell activation. Endothelial dysfunction is observed secondary to impaired nitric oxide release and increased vasoconstrictor formation such as thromboxane A2 as well as activation of the renin angiotensin system, exacerbating salt retention and ascites formation. Consequences can include hepatorenal syndrome and hepatopulmonary syndrome. Hepatic resistance to blood flow is noted resulting in portal hypertension, secondary to increased portal pressure. Portal pressure is worsened secondary to splanchnic vasodilation, leading to increased blood flow into the portal venous architecture. Portal hypertension is the primary factor for the development of varices, namely collateral branches and increased risk of bleeding. Shunting of portal blood into the systemic circulation via newly formed collateral branches results in hepatic encephalopathy secondary to reduced first pass metabolism and impaired ammonia detoxification.

Causes of cirrhosis are numerous and include excessive intake of alcohol, hepatitis B and C, autoimmune hepatitis, primary biliary cirrhosis, primary sclerosing cholangitis, haemochromatosis, Wilson's disease, alpha 1 antitrypsin deficiency, drugs such as methotrexate and amiodarone as well as venous outflow obstruction.

Symptoms
- Abdominal pain
- Confusion
- Fatigue

- Jaundice
- Haematemesis
- Melaena

Signs

- Abdominal distension secondary to ascites
- Hepatomegaly
- Encephalopathy (see Table 16 below)
- Signs of chronic liver disease (see examination section)
- Melaena

Table 16: West Haven Criteria: Signs/Symptoms

❑ Changes in behavior with minimal change in level of consciousness +1
❑ Gross disorientation, drowsiness, possibly asterixis, inappropriate behavior +2
❑ Marked confusion, incoherent speech, sleeping most of the time but arousable to vocal stimuli +3
❑ Comatose, unresponsive to pain; decorticate or decerebrate posturing +4

Differentials

- Budd Chiari syndrome
- Portal vein thrombosis
- Splenic vein thrombosis
- IVC obstruction
- Schistosomiasis

Investigations

Imaging is essential in such cases. Ultrasound/CT/MRI aids in the diagnosis of liver nodularity/evidence of portal hypertension. Transient elastography (FibroScan) is utilised to aid in determination of liver stiffness. Blood investigations are key and a full liver screen including clotting is required.

Management

Lifestyle advice should be offered to all patients, with emphasis on ceasing alcohol consumption and smoking if applicable. Obese patients should also be encouraged to lose weight as appropriate.

Treatment relies on the underlying cause: cause-specific treatments are discussed elsewhere in this book.

Patients with evidence of portal hypertension and varices require band ligation and the use of non-selective β blockers. Active bleeding requires appropriate resuscitation with band ligation, vasoactive drugs such as terlipressin, broad spectrum antibiotics and salvage therapies such as TIPS if unsuccessful.

Ascites requires sodium restriction, use of spironolactone and furosemide with paracentesis as needed.

Patients with evidence of encephalopathy benefit from lactulose and rifaximin.

Liver transplantation is utilised for those patients with decompensated disease (ascites, sepsis, bleeding, encephalopathy, non-obstructive jaundice) or the occurrence of hepatocellular carcinoma with cirrhosis. Further details on liver transplantation are highlighted in the examination section of this book.

Hereditary Haemochromatosis

Aetiopathogenesis

One of the most important components in hereditary haemochromatosis is the hormone hepcidin. This molecule helps to control the extracellular iron concentration through binding to and inducing the degradation of the iron exporter ferroportin. The loss of hepcidin is paramount to the occurrence of hereditary haemochromatosis as is genetic mutations such as HFE, TFR2, HAMP and HJV. The HFE gene is linked to iron transport but its exact role is still not concrete. Common mutations comprise the C282Y and H63D.

Symptoms
- Skin bronzing
- Joint pains
- Increased urinary frequency and thirst secondary to diabetes

Signs
- Hepatomegaly
- Hyperpigmentation
- Diabetes
- Arthropathy
- Amenorrhoea/impotence
- Cardiomyopathy
- Hair loss
- Koilonychia

Differentials

- Biliary cirrhosis
- Haemolytic anaemia

Investigations

Investigations of choice include measurement of the fasting transferrin saturation and serum ferritin. Those with increased transferrin saturation should undergo haemochromatosis gene (HFE) testing for C282Y and H63D polymorphisms. Patients may benefit from a chest X-ray and an echocardiogram in view of cardiomegaly-associated disease. It is important to note that a liver biopsy per se is not essential in making a diagnosis. Its use can be employed in C282Y homozygous patients with a serum ferritin greater than 1000 ug/l, elevated AST, hepatomegaly or those aged > 40 years.

In cases where C282Y homozygosity has been excluded, one must screen for alternative genetic mutations as mentioned above if there is evidence of iron excess on MRI/liver biopsy.

Management

Patients diagnosed with HFC haemochromatosis and excess iron should undergo phlebotomy. C282Y homozygotes without evidence of iron overload can be monitored on an annual basis and treated when ferritin exceeds normal limits. Phlebotomy should be performed weekly, removing approximately 500 ml of blood. It is important to ensure patients are screened for complications such as cirrhosis, diabetes, arthropathy, hypogonadism and porphyria cutanea tarda, and treated accordingly.

Wilson's Disease

Aetiopathogenesis

Wilson's disease has been attributed to dysfunction of the ATP7B gene responsible for the transmembrane transport of copper within hepatocytes. As a result, copper accumulates in the liver and eventually the blood stream, with dissemination in a multi-systemic fashion.

Symptoms

- Neurological e.g. tremor, dystonia, speaking difficulties, hand clumsiness, fits
- Psychiatric e.g. emotional lability, impulsiveness
- Symptoms secondary to anaemia
- Haematuria
- Joint pain

Signs

- Signs of chronic liver disease
- Neurological dysfunction e.g. ataxia, dystonia, mask-like facies
- Kayser Fleischer rings
- Anaemia
- Skeletal abnormalities

Differentials

- Acute liver failure
- Haemochromatosis
- Viral hepatitis

Investigations

Investigations of choice include those for serum ceruloplasmin (typically reduced), 24-hour urinary copper (>1.6 micromol), liver copper (> 4 micromol/g dry weight), presence of Coombs-negative haemolytic anaemia and mutation analysis. A MRI of the brain should be instigated in all cases of neurological Wilson's disease as well as an electrocardiogram to exclude cardiac-based manifestations. The Leipzig score establishes a positive diagnosis with a scoring of 4 or more and a likely diagnosis with a score of 3 or more (see Figure 7).

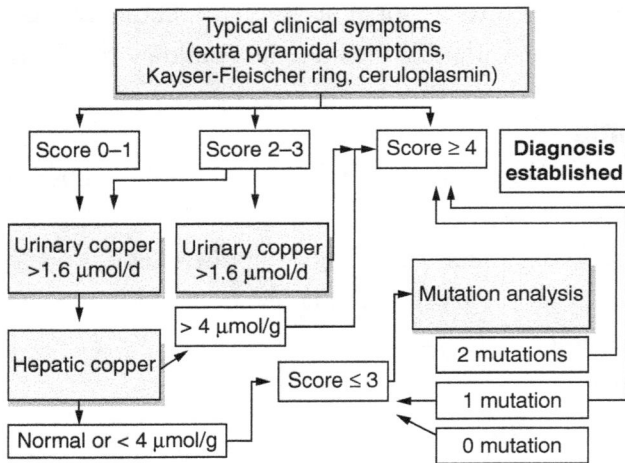

Fig. 7.   Leipzig scoring

Management

Management of Wilson's disease relies on a chelating agent, namely D penicillamine or trientine. Zinc has a potential role in neurological patients. Dietary therapy is key and patients should avoid copper-rich foods. Those patients acutely unresponsive to chelation therapy should be considered for liver transplantation.

Alpha-1 Antitrypsin Deficiency

Aetiopathogenesis

Alpha-1 antitrypsin (AAT) is a protease inhibitor with deficiency most frequently due to the SERPINA1 gene mutation. It is inherited in an autosomal codominant fashion with the ZZ genetic variant associated with a higher risk of liver disease, with MZ and SZ associated with a reduced risk. Evidence demonstrates that the Z protein forms polymers that trap AAT within the endoplasmic reticulum of hepatocytes, resulting in a reduction in AAT. As yet, it is not clear how such polymers may induce liver damage but an association is clearly evident.

Symptoms
- Symptoms are typically in line with those of acute liver failure/cirrhotic patients as highlighted previously

Signs
- Signs are in line with those of acute liver failure/cirrhosis as described previously

Differentials
- Viral hepatitis
- Autoimmune hepatitis
- Hepatocellular carcinoma
- Primary biliary cirrhosis
- Alcoholic hepatitis

- NAFLD
- Primary sclerosing cholangitis

Investigations

Investigations in this regard include serum AAT measurement and genotyping studies. A liver biopsy is generally not needed but can be considered to exclude other causes of liver disease.

Management

Treatment of AAT deficiency-related liver disease should follow the general management principles outlined for acute liver failure and cirrhosis discussed previously. Abstinence of alcohol is essential, with steps to avoid excessive weight gain. Liver transplantation should be considered as a curative form of treatment.

Autoimmune Hepatitis (AIH)

Aetiopathogenesis

Various viral agents have been implicated in the occurrence of AIH. Examples include measles, hepatitis, Cytomegalovirus and Epstein Barr. Drugs have also been implicated and comprise diclofenac, minocycline, methyldopa, nitrofurantoin and atorvastatin. From a genetic perspective, human leukocyte antigen (HLA) genes linked to chromosome 6 have been associated with the disease. Type 1 AIH is characterised by antinuclear antibodies, smooth muscle antibodies, anti-actin antibodies, pANCA and antibodies against soluble liver antigen and liver pancreas antigen. Type 2 AIH is linked with antibodies against liver kidney microsome 1 and liver cytosol 1. TNF alpha genetic associations is also noted with regard to AIH.

Final development of autoimmune damage is associated with decreased numbers of CD4 + CD25+ regulatory T cells.

Symptoms

- Fatigue
- Abdominal pain
- Pruritus
- Joint pain
- Skin rash
- Weight loss

Signs

- Hepatomegaly
- Jaundice

- Splenomegaly
- Ascites
- Encephalopathy
- Symptoms and signs secondary to associated autoimmune conditions may be present e.g. haematological or rheumatological

Differentials

- Viral hepatitis

Investigations

Investigations of choice are shown in Table 17.

Table 17:

Features	Definite AIH
Liver histology	Interface hepatitis of moderate or severe activity with or without lobular hepatitis or bridging necrosis. No biliary lesions, granulomas or other prominent changes suggestive of a different aetiology.
Laboratory features	Any serum aminotransferase abnormality, especially if alkaline phosphatase activity normal. Normal levels of alpha-1 antitrypsin, copper and caeruloplasmin.
Serum immunoglobulins	Globulin, γ-globulin or IgG concentrations >1.5 × upper normal limit.
Serum autoantibodies	ANA, SMA or anti-LKM-1 antibodies at titres ≥ 1:80. Lower titres acceptable for children, especially anti-LKM-1. Negative AMA.

Imaging investigations are worthwhile and include an abdominal ultrasound scan/CT.

Management

Initial treatment of choice relies on prednisolone in addition to azathioprine. Alternative therapy in non-responders includes tacrolimus. In patients with liver failure, bridging necrosis on liver biopsy or jaundiced patients with a poorly improving MELD score, transplantation should be considered.

In view of steroid treatment, patients should be commenced on calcium and vitamin D supplementation with DEXA scanning-based investigations. It is important to note that those patients intolerant of azathioprine require treatment with mycophenolate mofetil (MMF).

Primary Biliary Cirrhosis (PBC)

Aetiopathogenesis

Various factors account for the occurrence of PBC, and these include a genetic association comprising polymorphisms of STAT4 and IL12A. Environmental factors are also key and comprise bacterial links such as *Escherichia coli* and *Novosphingobium aromaticivorans*.

It has been known for some time that the condition is essentially autoimmune in nature and linked, to loss of immune tolerance to self-mitochondrial proteins. In addition, research demonstrates the existence of autoreactive CD8 and CD4 + T cells to the E2 aspect of the pyruvate dehydrogenase complex in addition to reduced numbers of regulatory T cells (which help to prevent autoreactivity). The end result is apoptotic damage to biliary epithelium.

Symptoms

- Fatigue
- Pruritus secondary to bile deposition in the skin
- Abdominal pain

Signs

- Hepatomegaly
- Splenomegaly
- Jaundice
- Xanthelasmata
- Sicca syndrome

Differentials

- AIH
- Biliary obstruction
- Primary sclerosing cholangitis

Investigations

Patients should undergo initial LFTs to assess the existence of an elevated alkaline phosphatase (ALP). An ultrasound is important and can demonstrate the presence of dilated bile ducts or a focal lesion. Antibody screening for AMA/AMA type M2 is strongly suggestive of the diagnosis. If antibody screening is negative, patients should proceed for liver biopsy +/− MRCP/endoscopic ultrasound. Additional findings may include an abnormal lipid profile and a raised ESR.

Management

Initial treatment relies on ursodeoxycholic acid (UDCA) long term. Those with a poor response to UDCA may benefit from a combination of UDCA and budesonide. In strongly advanced disease (namely a bilirubin >103 micromol/l or decompensated cirrhosis), patients should be referred for liver transplantation.

Primary Sclerosing Cholangitis (PSC)

Aetiopathogenesis

PSC is linked to the occurrence of toxic bile acid metabolites, as well as potential viral infections. It was once assumed that bacteria were associated with the disease, yet antibiotics have no role in hindering progression. Genetic factors are implicated and include an association with HLA B8 and DR 3. Immune-related occurrences include the upregulation of lymphocytes, an increase in IgM, pANCA and complement. Such a response helps to explain the association with inflammatory bowel disease. There is also a decrease in the number of T cells in the circulation with an increase in the number of B cells and enhanced auto-reactivity of portal T lymphocytes leading to inflammation and eventually scarring of intra- and extra-hepatic bile ducts.

Symptoms
- Fatigue
- Jaundice
- Pruritus
- Abdominal pain

Signs
- Signs typical of acute/chronic liver failure

Investigations

Evidence of cholestasis from initial LFTs is key in making a diagnosis. In addition, patients can benefit from a liver biopsy and ERCP/MRCP/percutaneous transhepatic cholangiography.

Management

Treatment relies on UDCA which has been shown to improve LFTs but not survival. Steroids and other immunosuppressants are typically instigated in cases of overlap syndrome. Biliary strictures should be treated with dilatation and appropriate antibiotic coverage. End-stage disease requires liver transplantation.

Liver Abscess

Aetiopathogenesis

Two primary forms of liver abscess exist, pyogenic and amoebic. Pyogenic liver abscesses occur typically due to cholangitis secondary to stones or strictures, abdominal infection as seen in cases of diverticulitis, Crohn's disease, appendicitis or perforated peptic ulcer disease or endocarditis. Infective organisms comprise *Escherichia coli*, *Klebsiella pneumoniae*, *Bacteroides*, *Staphylococci* and *Streptococcus*. Immunosuppression as seen in acquired immune deficiency syndrome (AIDS), drug use such as in chemotherapy and transplantation are also accountable.

Amoebic liver abscesses are secondary to the parasite *Entamoeba histolytica*, which is transmitted via the faecal-oral route. Within the small intestine the cyst wall disintegrates leading to the release of trophozoites. Migration to the large bowel and liver follows with abscess formation typically affecting the right lobe, comprising anchovy paste-type necrotic tissue.

Symptoms

- Abdominal pain
- Cough
- Dyspnoea
- Pleuritic chest pain
- Fever
- Sweats
- Vomiting
- Weight loss
- Diarrhoea in the case of an amoebic liver abscess

Signs

- Hepatomegaly
- Abdominal tenderness
- Jaundice
- Pleural rub
- Reduced breath sounds in case of pleural effusion

Differentials

- Cholecystitis
- Hepatocellular carcinoma
- Hydatid cyst

Investigations

Investigations of choice include a FBC which may show evidence of anaemia of chronic disease as well as a raised white cell count. LFTs typically demonstrate a raised alkaline phosphatase with abnormal trans-aminase levels and bilirubin. An abdominal and chest X-ray should be requested which may demonstrate evidence of hepatomegaly with an air fluid level as well as a raised hemidiaphragm/pleural effusion. An abdominal ultrasound/CT scan should be utilised to determine stronger evidence of abscess formation. Stool analysis may help to identify cysts in the case of amoebic liver abscesses. Serology and serum antigen testing for *E histolytica* is also advised.

Management

Pyogenic liver abscesses should be treated with antibiotics such as penicillin, an aminoglycoside, metronidazole, or third-generation cephalosporin. In addition to antibiotics, patients should undergo drainage.

Amoebic liver abscesses should be treated with metronidazole in the first instance. Diloxanide furoate aids in the elimination of intestinal amoebae. Drainage should take place if the abscess is extensive in size, patients have not responded appropriately to antibiotics or if rupture is likely.

Budd Chiari Syndrome (BCS)

Aetiopathogenesis

The underlying aetiopathogenesis of BCS is secondary to hepatic venous outflow obstruction and subsequent portal hypertension with possible thrombosis. The end result is hypoxic hepatocyte damage and necrosis, with eventual fibrosis and cirrhosis formation. Causes of BCS include hypercoagulable states such as antithrombin III deficiency, myeloproliferative disease, malignancy, pregnancy and the antiphospholipid syndrome as well as the oral contraceptive pill.

Symptoms

- Abdominal pain
- Ascites
- Nausea
- Jaundice
- Confusion in view of possible encephalopathy

Signs

- Jaundice
- Hepatomegaly
- Ascites
- Abdominal tenderness

Differentials

- Appendicitis
- Pancreatitis

- Biliary atresia
- Viral hepatitis
- NAFLD
- Congestive cardiac failure

Investigations

Investigations of choice include a FBC and LFTs which will demonstrate evidence of abnormal aminotransferase levels as well as a rise in alkaline phosphatase and bilirubin. Analysis of the serum-ascitic fluid albumin gradient demonstrates a notable rise.

Imaging tools comprise Doppler ultrasound as well as CT/MRI to highlight evidence of necrosis and occlusion. Evidence of a 'spider-web'-like pattern on venography is diagnostic.

Management

Management of BCS relies on ascitic drainage and use of diuretics, with albumin infusion as appropriate. Anticoagulation with warfarin is advised in the long term with initial use of heparin. Acute cases of BCS require thrombolysis with urokinase or tissue plasminogen activator. In the case of inferior vena cava (IVC) webs/stenosis or focal hepatic vein stenosis, patients should undergo angioplasty +/− stenting. Acute cases of BCS require TIPS intervention with surgical shunts if the portocaval pressure gradient is >10 mm Hg. Intervention courtesy of transplantation is undertaken in cases of fulminant BCS, existence of cirrhosis or failure of shunt insertion.

Hepatocellular Carcinoma (HCC)

Aetiopathogenesis

HCC (or, more commonly, liver cancer) typically occurs secondary to risk factors such as Hepatitis B, Hepatitis C, alcoholic liver disease and NAFLD. Often these risk factors induce cirrhosis which later leads to HCC. Additional causes include smoking and excessive alcohol as well as the mycotoxin aflatoxin and a history of diabetes. Pathogenesis-wise, mutations of importance include TP53, CTNNB1 (the gene for β catenin) and PTEN. Oncogenic activation has been shown to occur, namely of MYC. Proliferation cascades are activated and include EGFR and Ras. Angiogenesis occurs courtesy of VEGF A and fibroblast growth factor signalling.

Symptoms
- Fever
- Weight loss
- Abdominal pain
- Jaundice
- Loss of appetite
- Nausea and vomiting

Signs
- Hepatomegaly
- Signs of chronic liver disease

Differentials

- Cholangiocarcinoma
- Focal nodular hyperplasia
- Liver cyst
- Haemangioma
- Fibroma

Investigations

Investigations comprise a FBC (to exclude anaemia and thrombocytopenia/cytosis), U and E's (to exclude evidence of hyponatremia and hypercalcaemia), LFTs, coagulation profile, serum glucose (typically reduced), hepatitis serology, AFP, alpha-1 antitrypsin level and iron studies. Imaging is usually in the form of an abdominal ultrasound/CT or MRI.

Management

European Association for the Study of the Liver (EASL) guidelines suggest the first-line treatment as surgery for patients with solitary tumours, a normal bilirubin, platelet count > 100,000/mm^3 and hepatic venous pressure gradient < 10 mm Hg. Liver transplantation is undertaken in cases of single tumours < 5 cm or < 3 nodules < 3 cm.

Ablation with radiofrequency or percutaneous ethanol injection is advised for those with Barcelona clinic liver cancer 0-A tumours not suitable for surgery.

Chemoembolisation is advised in those with BCLC stage B. Sorafenib is the standard therapy for HCC, preferred for those with well-preserved liver function and with advanced tumours e.g. BCLC C. For those with bone metastases, radiotherapy is useful. BCLC D-stage patients require palliative care input alongside. It is important to note that such patients also require pain and nutritional support.

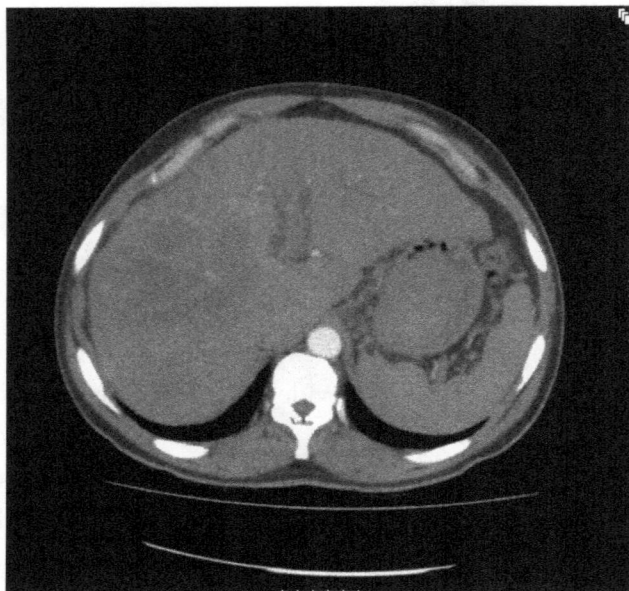

Fig. 8.   Evidence of an enlarged cirrhotic liver with hepatocellular carcinoma occupying the right liver lobe

Common Bile Duct Stones

Aetiopathogenesis

Gallstones are crystalline-based deposits, usually cholesterol, pigment, calcium or a mixture of these in nature. Factors responsible for the formation of gallstones include excessive bile cholesterol, low bile salts, and reduced gallbladder motility. Risk factors specific for cholesterol stone formation include female gender, pregnancy, high oestrogen levels, drugs such as fibrates and somatostatin analogues, increasing age, ethnicity, obesity and conditions such as cirrhosis and IBD. Pigment stones are formed courtesy of haemolysis as seen in sickle cell anaemia for example, and bacterial-based infection.

Symptoms

- Right upper quadrant abdominal pain

(It is important to note that patients may be asymptomatic)

Signs

- Abdominal tenderness/guarding
- Jaundice

Differentials

- Pancreatitis
- Peptic ulcer disease
- Cholangiocarcinoma
- Appendicitis

Investigations

Investigations of choice include a FBC and LFTs (which may demonstrate an obstructive picture or hepatitis) in addition to a coagulation screen. Imaging in the first instance comprises an ultrasound scan, in addition to an endoscopic ultrasound (EUS)/MRI.

Management

Management can rely on stone extraction courtesy of an ERCP. It is important to take note of any coagulation abnormality and correct accordingly. Adequate drainage is essential for those patients with common bile duct stones that have not been successfully extracted. Therefore the interim use of stents is advised prior to a repeat ERCP. Alternative treatment comprises surgical intervention in the form of laparoscopic cholecystectomy. For those not suitable for surgery, extra corporeal shock wave lithotripsy is a suitable alternative.

Acute Cholecystitis

Aetiopathogenesis

Acute cholecystitis is associated with obstruction of the cystic duct or neck of the gallbladder by gallstones or biliary sludge. Cystic duct obstruction leads to increased intraluminal pressure within the gall-bladder and along with cholesterol-rich bile, triggers an inflammatory response secondary to prostaglandin I and E2. Bacterial organisms dominate and include *E coli*, *Klebsiella* and *S faecalis*.

Symptoms

- Right upper quadrant abdominal pain
- Nausea
- Vomiting

Signs

- Fever
- Murphy's sign, namely inhibition of inspiration on palpation
- Guarding/rebound tenderness
- Jaundice (typically uncommon). Note the triad of fever, right upper quadrant pain and jaundice usually implies cholangitis

Differentials

- Abdominal aortic aneurysm
- Acute mesenteric ischaemia
- Cholangiocarcinoma

- Cholangitis
- Peptic ulcer disease
- Pyelonephritis

Investigations

Blood investigations should be performed and include a FBC to exclude infection, U and E's and LFTs. An amylase should be requested to exclude pancreatitis and a urine screen to exclude pyelonephritis. Abdominal ultrasound scanning/CT/MRI are initial investigations of choice which may demonstrate evidence of an oedematous gallbladder/ wall thickening/gallstone presence. The gold standard investigation of choice is biliary scintigraphy (hydroxyiminodiacetic acid (HIDA) scan). In patients with acute cholecystitis the gallbladder will not show any evidence of HIDA up to two hours after injection.

Management

Management relies on appropriate fluid resuscitation, analgesia, anti-inflammatory agents and antibiotic therapy such as piperacillin/ tazobactam, meropenem, metronidazole or a cephalosporin. Surgical cholecystectomy intervention is typically undertaken laparoscopically.

A percutaneous cholecystostomy is indicated in high-risk surgical patients.

Acute Pancreatitis

Aetiopathogenesis

Acute pancreatitis is thought to occur secondary to trypsin activation within the acinar cells in addition to the formation of trypsin inhibitors such as SPINK1. This results in gland autodigestion and inflammation. The main causes of such a disorder comprise gallstones and excessive alcohol. In addition to trypsin activation, elastase and phospholipase A2 are upregulated. Inflammation can occur secondary to the formation of IL1, IL6 and IL8. The production of oxygen free radicals also results in significant injury.

Symptoms

- Abdominal pain often radiating to the back
- Nausea and vomiting
- Anorexia
- Diarrhoea

Signs

- Fever
- Haemodynamic instability
- Abdominal tenderness/guarding/rigidity
- Absent bowel sounds
- Jaundice
- Cullen's sign

- Grey Turner's sign
- Purtscher's retinopathy

Differentials

- Acute mesenteric ischaemia
- Cholangitis
- Cholecystitis
- Chronic pancreatitis
- Peptic ulcer disease
- Pancreatic cancer

Investigations

Recommended investigations include a serum amylase and lipase in addition to an abdominal ultrasound/CT scan. An EUS may be helpful in cases of microlithiasis. Other worthwhile investigations include a

Table 18:   Features that may predict a severe attack of acute pancreatitis, present within 48 hours of admission to hospital

Initial assessment	Clinical impression of severity Body mass index > 30 Pleural effusion on chest radiograph APACHE II score > 8
24 hours after admission	Clinical impression of severity APACHE II score > 8 Glasgow score 3 or more Persisting organ failure, especially if multiple C reactive protein > 150 mg/l
48 hours after admission	Clinical impression of severity Glasgow score 3 or more C reactive protein > 150 mg/l Persisting organ failure for 48 hours Multiple or progressive organ failure

Modified from the World Association guidelines.

Table 19:   Computed tomography (CT) grading of severity of acute pancreatitis

CT grade	
(A) Normal pancreas	0
(B) Oedematous pancreatitis	1
(C) B plus mild extrapancreatic changes	2
(D) Severe extrapancreatic changes including one fluid collection	3
(E) Multiple or extensive extrapancreatic collections	4
Necrosis	
None	0
< One third	2
> One third, < one half	4
> Half	6
CT severity index = CT grade + necrosis score	
	Complications
0–3	8%
4–6	35%
7–10	92%
	Deaths
0–3	3%
4–6	6%
7–10	17%

Modified from the World Association guidelines and based on Balthazar and colleagues.

MRCP in suspected duct obstruction and an ERCP which has therapeutic potential in terms of stone extraction. LFTs are recommended in cases of suspected gallstone pancreatitis. Additional investigations include U and E's, serum glucose (typically elevated) and serum calcium (often elevated) and a lipid profile. A FBC will help to determine

Table 20: Ranson's criteria for mortality risk of acute pancreatitis (Estimates mortality of patients with pancreatitis, based on initial and 48-hour lab values)

On Admission	
WBC > 16k on admission	+1 YES 0 NO
Age > 55	+1 YES 0 NO
Glucose > 200mg/dL (> 10 mmol/L) on admission	+1 YES 0 NO
AST > 250 on admission	+1 YES 0 NO
LDH > 350 on admission	+1 YES 0 NO
48 Hours into Admission	
Hct drop > 10% from admission	+1 YES 0 NO
BUN increase > 5mg/dL (> 1.79 mmol/L) from admission	+1 YES 0 NO
Ca < 8 mg/dL (< 2 mmol/L) within 48 hours	+1 YES 0 NO
Arterial pO2 < 60 mmHg within 48 hours	+1 YES 0 NO
Base deficit (24 - HCO3) > 4 mg/dL within 48 hours	+1 YES 0 NO
Fluid needs > 6L within 48 hours	+1 YES 0 NO

evidence of sepsis in addition to a CRP. An arterial blood gas helps to determine one's lactate and oxygenation levels. This investigation is particularly important in cases of suspected acute respiratory distress syndrome (ARDS).

Management

According to the British Society of Gastroenterology (BSG), antibiotic use is not so clear-cut. Antibiotics recommended include imipenem, metronidazole and cefuroxime. Feeding is also recommended and should typically be enterally. If gallstones are the suspected cause, then patients should undergo an ERCP within 72 hours. A definitive plan for cholecystectomy should also be made once over the acute phase to prevent recurrence of an attack. Patients with persistent symptoms and greater than 30% necrosis along with sepsis should undergo fine needle aspiration (FNA) for culture. Infected necrosis requires intervention to help debride all necrotic tissue. And it goes without saying that such cases should be managed ideally in an intensive therapy unit (ITU) setting.

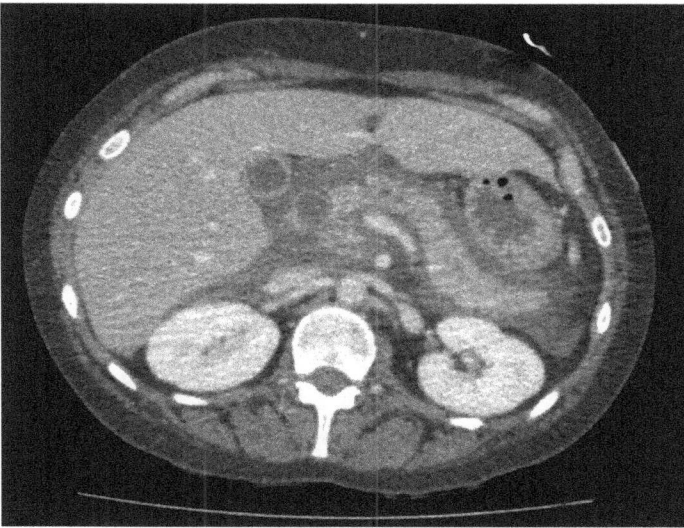

Fig. 9.   Abdominal CT demonstrating evidence of free fluid, gallstones and inflammatory changes in the pancreas in keeping with acute pancreatitis

Chronic Pancreatitis

Aetiopathogenesis

Chronic pancreatitis has been attributed to the initial occurrence of pancreastasis, which is triggered by reactive oxygen species (ROS). In addition, there is an increase in enzyme and calcium production with a decrease in the protease inhibitor SPINK 1 and bicarbonate. Production of stress proteins such as pancreatitis-associated protein (PAP) and pancreatic stone protein (PSP) takes place as well as GP-2, a component of zymogen granule membranes. Overexpression of cytochrome P450 enzymes is also noted. Chronic pancreatitis is also triggered by stellate cell activation and subsequent fibrosis. Causes of chronic pancreatitis include excessive alcohol, smoking, drugs such as azathioprine and sodium valproate, hyperlipidaemia and hypercalcaemia, genetic factors such as cystic fibrosis transmembrane conductance regulator (CFTR) mutations as well as gallstones and autoimmune causes.

Symptoms
- Abdominal pain which may radiate to the back
- Diarrhoea
- Weight loss

Signs
- Abdominal tenderness or discomfort
- Evidence of muscle wasting

Differentials

- Cholangitis
- IBD
- PUD
- Pancreatic cancer

Investigations

Investigations of choice comprise serum amylase and lipase (typically elevated in acute attacks, however), faecal elastase (200 microg/g stool is deemed normal), an abdominal X-ray (demonstrating evidence of calcification) and CT scan, ERCP (for ductal system analysis)/MRCP (for assessment of ductal system and parenchyma) as well as EUS (to determine the presence of cysts, lobularity, duct dilatation and hyperechoic foci, for example). It is also worthwhile testing serum calcium levels to ascertain an underlying cause.

Management

Chronic pancreatitis patients should be offered endocrine (insulin) and exocrine (pancreatic enzymes, namely Creon) replacement therapies as well as adequate analgesia. Endoscopic therapies can include treatment for duct stenosis, strictures and stones. Those suitable for surgery can benefit from either partial or total pancreatectomy or pancreatic duct drainage. Pain management may rely on splanchnicectomy through an EUS approach or radiofrequency ablation.

TOPIC

Pancreatic Cancer

Aetiopathogenesis

The causes of pancreatic cancer include smoking, excessive alcohol and coffee intake and a background of chronic pancreatitis. Pathogenesis-wise, the condition arises first as pancreatic intraepithelial neoplasia, progressing eventually to invasive carcinoma. This process is governed by activation of the KRAS2 oncogene as well as inactivation of the tumour suppressor genes CDKN2A, TP53 and DPC4. The development of pancreatic cancer is associated with the occurrence of a desmoplastic reaction courtesy of stellate cells, activated by growth factors. Such cells are also linked to impaired vascularisation associated with the condition.

Symptoms

- Abdominal pain with radiation to the back
- Nausea
- Fatigue
- Diarrhoea secondary to malabsorption
- Weight loss secondary to anorexia and malabsorption
- Jaundice with darkening of urine/paler stools in pancreatic head carcinoma
- Pruritus

Signs

- Epigastric pain
- Palpable abdominal mass
- Ascites

- Sister Mary Joseph nodules (subcutaneous metastases in the para-umbilical area)
- Migratory thrombophlebitis
- Cervical lymphadenopathy

Differentials

- Acute/chronic pancreatitis
- Cholangitis
- Cholecystitis
- PUD
- Gastric cancer

Investigations

Investigations of choice include an abdominal ultrasound/CT/ERCP/MRCP. EUS is also a useful investigative tool. PET scanning is often employed to image the primary tumour and evidence of metastases. A tissue sample is essential in confirming a diagnosis. Tumour markers which are elevated in cases of pancreatic cancer include CA 19-9 and CEA. Blood investigations include a FBC (which will often demonstrate evidence of anaemia and thrombocytosis) in addition to a rise in bilirubin and ALP in cases of obstructive jaundice. Patients may demonstrate evidence of an elevated amylase and lipase as well as a low serum albumin secondary to malnutrition.

Management

Many patients require relief of obstructive jaundice by placement of a plastic stent. A surgical bypass is preferred in those who are likely to survive six months. Any form of duodenal obstruction should be treated surgically.

Endoscopic stent placement is the preferred option as opposed to transhepatic stenting. If endoscopic stent placement fails, percutaneous placement of a self-expanding metal stent is the next option of choice.

If a stent is placed prior to surgery, this should be plastic in nature and placed endoscopically.

In terms of surgery, pancreaticoduodenectomy is the most appropriate resection intervention for pancreatic head tumours. Left-sided resection with splenectomy is suited for localised carcinomas of the body and tail of the pancreas.

A duodenal bypass is employed during palliative surgery. Non-surgical therapies for palliation comprise chemotherapy, namely gemcitabine. Pain relief is typically via the World Health Organisation (WHO) analgesic ladder and palliative care input. In addition, patients may benefit from neurolytic coeliac plexus block, chemoradiation and pancreatic enzyme supplements.

Examination Skills

Introduction

Effective examination skills are key to determining a diagnosis alongside an accurate history. During medical school and early junior doctor years, the assessment of examination skills during an OSCE or postgraduate examination setting is something feared by most, if not all. Regardless of this fact, it is important to note that there are only a finite number of stations that can appear. What you must remember is that the mark schemes at either an undergraduate/postgraduate level are universal. Examiners are expecting you to demonstrate an appropriate rapport with the patient in the first instance, being mindful of any concerns they may have during the examination. In addition, candidates should be able to perform a thorough and systematic systems examination and be prepared to detect physical signs, construct differentials and detail potential investigation and management strategies. Each station is schema-dependent, so be wary of preferred presentation style. For example, an examiner may simply ask you to palpate the abdomen. In addition, some may prefer you not to talk through your examination as you perform it. You can imagine how laborious it becomes for them when the candidate begins as follows: *I am standing at the end of the bed and observing for any scars or masses... I am now looking at the hands for clubbing* ... It may seem that they are rushing you through but that is so they can reach all station aspects and ensure you can gain as many points as possible.

The following cases are all likely at an undergraduate and postgraduate level, some harder than others. However, if faced with difficulty, keep things simple and DO NOT invent signs. Examiners are quick to spot the actor-type candidate and this will not bode well in terms of professionalism/probity. Be observant of the fact that you are only likely to face a 2–3-minute interplay with the examiner post-examination, so follow the pattern of signs, differentials, investigations and management and make sure to keep it sharp and, most of all, simple. Examiners get frustrated with long-drawn out negatives and several random causes which are not applicable to pathology in the UK. In other words, an opening discussion could be something along the following lines… *On examination the patient appears comfortable/distressed. There is evidence of x, y and z. The most likely diagnosis is… secondary to x, y and z.*

Or

I am unsure of the diagnosis but would like to offer the following differentials. In order to obtain a diagnosis I would undertake the following tests.

Start with blood investigations before imaging. And if you are 100% convinced of the diagnosis, then offer a management plan. OK, on to the cases!

The Liver

Signs

You are highly unlikely to get an acutely unwell liver case as such cases are bound to be intubated in ITU, so try not to invent exaggerated grades of encephalopathy! Remember to look for potential chronic liver disease signs, namely jaundice, ascites (detail evidence of an everted umbilicus, dullness to percussion, shifting dullness), clubbing, palmar erythema, spider naevi, bruising (due to impaired coagulation), gynecomastia (due to excess oestrogen), caput medusae (abdominal wall vein prominence), hepatomegaly, splenomegaly or both (due to portal hypertension), oedema (secondary to hypoalbuminaemia) and muscle wasting.

When presenting evidence of an enlarged liver, detail the distance in cm below the level of the coastal margin, evidence of tenderness, surface hardness, nodularity and presence of a bruit. One essential sign is to assess for the presence of asterixis or flapping tremor of the outstretched hands.

Differentials

Differentials are numerous for a chronic liver disease patient. And include cirrhosis secondary to, say, alcohol, infective causes such as hepatitis B and C, autoimmune causes, primary biliary cirrhosis/sclerosing cholangitis, haemochromatosis, Wilson's disease and drugs such as methotrexate and amiodarone. Remember that additional causes of hepatomegaly include malignancy, right heart failure, abscesses and infiltration such as is the case with amyloidosis.

Investigations

For chronic liver disease, investigations under the acute liver failure section still apply. In addition, appropriate ascites investigations are essential (see previous section).

Management

And so next is the question of management. In a broad sense you would determine the underlying cause. If alcohol excess is a problem, then abstinence is key. Again, refer to the sections on ascites and relevant causes described previously. There may be a discussion on liver transplantation and hence it is important to have some understanding of this topic.

According to the BSG, absolute and relative contraindications to liver transplantation include the following:

Absolute Contraindications

AIDS
Extrahepatic malignancy
Advanced cardiopulmonary disease
Cholangiocarcinoma

Relative Contraindications

HIV positivity
Age above 70 years
Significant sepsis outside the extrahepatic biliary tree
HBV DNA positivity
Active alcohol/substance misuse
Severe psychiatric disorder
Portal venous system thrombosis
Pulmonary hypertension

Some important pointers for referral depending on condition:

- PBC — Serum bilirubin >100 micromol/l
- PSC — Childs Pugh score C
- ALD — A six-month abstinence period is desirable
- Hepatitis B — patients must be HBV DNA-negative prior to transplantation
- Hepatitis C — genotype and viral load should not influence transplant assessment
- HCC — see previous section

The Spleen

Signs

Splenomegaly is another common case encountered in an abdominal examination. And it is often tricky to distinguish between an enlarged spleen and an enlarged kidney. Important signs to look for include anaemia, co-existing evidence of chronic liver disease, lymphadenopathy in view of malignancy and rheumatological signs if concerned about the possibility of Felty's syndrome (rheumatoid arthritis, splenomegaly and neutropenia). Detail evidence of splenic enlargement x cm below the left costal margin and enlargement in the direction of the right iliac fossa. Describe whether there is dullness to percussion and existence of a splenic bruit which implies vascular congestion.

Differentials

- Spherocytosis
- Thalassemia major
- Splenic vein thrombosis
- Portal hypertension
- Sarcoidosis
- Malignancy e.g. chronic lymphocytic leukaemia (CLL)/chronic myeloid leukaemia (CML)
- Infective e.g. Epstein-Barr Virus/Malaria
- Autoimmune e.g. rheumatoid arthritis

Investigations

Blood investigations are an initial first step to exclude the presence of anaemia, leukopenia and thrombocytopenia. Imaging in the form of an ultrasound/CT is beneficial as well as a lymph node/bone marrow biopsy.

Management

Management is cause-dependent with chemotherapy for haematological malignancies and immunosuppression for autoimmune disease, for example. A splenectomy is performed in cases such as spherocytosis or immune thrombocytopenic purpura (ITP). Overwhelming post-splenectomy infection (OPSI) is common, and prevention of an occurrence involves appropriate treatment against *S pneumoniae*, *H influenzae* type B and *meningococci*.

The Kidneys

Signs

The main stations encountered here include those patients on renal replacement therapy (RRT) and polycystic kidney disease. For RRT, look for access e.g. a central venous catheter, arterio venous fistula or peritoneal catheter. Comment on the access site and existence of infection. It is important to look for scars in either the right or left iliac fossa for evidence of a transplanted kidney. Detail size, tenderness and feel, as well as the existence of a bruit. Additional signs to look for in any chronic kidney disease patient include asterixis due to uraemia and a pericardial rub secondary to uraemic pericarditis. Determine whether the patient appears anaemic and whether there is any evidence of immunosuppressive therapy ongoing e.g. bruising in the case of steroids or a Cushing-type appearance. Determine the patient's blood pressure if time allows and inform the examiner you will undertake a urinalysis for the existence of blood and protein.

Differentials

- Polycystic kidney disease
- Glomerulonephritis
- Diabetic nephropathy
- Multiple myeloma
- Hypertensive nephropathy

Investigations

Blood investigations, including a FBC and U and E's are a good first step, as well as a urinalysis. Undertaking a bone profile is important to exclude the presence of renal bone disease. Additional tests comprise urine and protein electrophoresis to exclude myeloma, an autoimmune screen, anti-GBM antibodies to exclude Goodpasture syndrome and imaging in the form of an ultrasound scan/CT. When the diagnosis is unclear, a renal biopsy should be undertaken.

Management

Management involves treatment of the underlying cause in addition to adequate blood pressure control, treatment of hyperlipidaemia and hyperglycaemia. Nephrotoxic drugs such as NSAIDs should be stopped and patients with proteinuria should be commenced on angiotensin-converting enzyme (ACE) inhibitors. Anaemia should be treated once an Hb of < 10 g/dl is reached with epoetin, hyperphosphataemia should be managed with phosphate binders, and calcium should be replaced if low. For patients with evidence of metabolic acidosis, sodium bicarbonate can be commenced and volume overload should be treated with diuretics.

You may be questioned on the indications for RRT. These include severe metabolic acidosis, hyperkalaemia, pericarditis, encephalopathy, refractory volume overload and peripheral neuropathy. In all cases, a GFR of 5–9 ml/min/1.73 m^2 is a requirement for RRT. Dietary measures are important and include a reduction in both protein and salt.

Examiners may also ask you the potential complications of RRT:

- Haemodialysis — cardiac compromise, air embolism, sepsis, mechanical obstruction of catheter or fistula, metabolic disturbance and amyloid deposition
- Peritoneal dialysis — cardiac compromise, infection at catheter site, mechanical obstruction as well as metabolic abnormalities.

Highlighted Case — Polycystic Kidney Disease (PKD)

Signs

PKD presents as bilateral flank masses. Evidence of chronic liver disease (secondary to polycystic liver disease) should be looked for as well as the existence of anaemia and hypertension. Observe for nephrectomy scars secondary to haemorrhage, for example. You may inform the examiner you would like to assess for the existence of a mitral valve prolapse or aortic regurgitation in addition to a third nerve palsy.

Differentials

- Cystic disease of the kidney
- Von Hippel Lindau disease

Investigations

In addition to the investigations detailed above, PKD patients should undergo genetic testing for autosomal dominant polycystic kidney disease (ADPKD) mutations and magnetic resonance angiography to exclude intracranial aneurysms.

Management

Management relies on the general measures described above in addition to pain control and surgical intervention in the case of an infected renal or hepatic cyst.

References

Adams PC, Barton JC. Haemochromatosis. *Lancet*. 1 Dec 2007; 370(9602): 1855–1860.

AGA technical review on the evaluation and management of chronic diarrhea. *Gastroenterology*. 1999; 116: 1464–1486.

Allum WH, Blazeby JM, Griffin SM, *et al*. Association of Upper Gastrointestinal Surgeons of Great Britain and Ireland; British Society of Gastroenterology; British Association of Surgical Oncology. Guidelines for the management of oesophageal and gastric cancer. *Gut*. Nov 2011; 60(11): 1449–1472.

American Association for the Study of Liver Diseases. Acute liver failure. AASLD practice guidelines. Available from http://www.aasld.org/publications/practice-guidelines-0.

Angulo P. Nonalcoholic fatty liver disease. *N Engl J Med*. 18 Apr 2002; 346(16): 1221–1231.

Baumgart DC, Carding SR. Inflammatory bowel disease: Cause and immunobiology. *Lancet*. 12 May 2007; 369(9573): 1627–1640.

Beggs AD, Latchford AR, Vasen HF, *et al*. Peutz-Jeghers syndrome: A systematic review and recommendations for management. *Gut*. Jul 2010; 59(7): 975–986.

Bernal W, Auzinger G, Dhawan A, Wendon J. Acute liver failure. *Lancet*. 17 Jul 2010; 376(9736): 190–201.

Blencowe NS, Strong S, Hollowood AD. Spontaneous oesophageal rupture. *BMJ*. 2013; 346.

Booth JCL, O'Grady J, Neuberger J. Royal College of Physicians of London; British Society of Gastroenterology. Clinical guidelines on the management of hepatitis C. *Gut*. Jul 2001; 49 Suppl 1: 11–21.

Braganza JM, Lee SH, McCloy RF, McMahon MJ. Chronic pancreatitis. *Lancet*. 2 Apr 2011; 377(9772): 1184–1197.

Bredenoord AJ, Pandolfino JE, Smout AJ. Gastro-oesophageal reflux disease. *Lancet.* 1 Jun 2013; 381(9881): 1933–1942.

Brenner H, Kloor M, Pox CP. Colorectal cancer. *Lancet.* 26 Apr 2014; 383(9927): 1490–1502.

British Society of Gastroenterology. Chronic management: Chronic pancreatitis. Available from http://www.bsg.org.uk/clinical/commissioning-report/chronic-pancreatitis.html.

British Society of Gastroenterology. Chronic management: NASH and non-alcoholic fatty liver disease. Available from http://www.bsg.org.uk/clinical/commissioning-report/nash-and-non-alcoholic-fatty-liver-disease.html.

Ciclitira PJ, Dewar DH, McLaughlin SD, Sanders DS. British Society of Gastroenterology. The management of adults with coeliac disease. Available from http://www.bsg.org.uk/images/stories/clinical/bsg_coeliac_10.pdf.

Devlin J, O'Grady J. Indications for referral and assessment in adult liver transplantation: A clinical guideline. *Gut.* Dec 1999; 45 Suppl 6: vi1–vi22.

Di Sabatino A, Corazza GR. Coeliac disease. *Lancet.* 25 Apr 2009; 373(9673): 1480–1493.

Drossman DA, Camilleri M, Mayer EA, *et al.* AGA technical review on irritable bowel syndrome. *Gastroenterology.* December 2002; 123(6): 2108–2131.

EASL-EORTC Clinical practice guidelines: Management of hepatocellular carcinoma. Available from http://www.easl.eu/research/our-contributions/clinical-practice-guidelines/detail/easl-eortc-clinical-practice-guidelines-Management-of-hepatocellular-carcinoma.

El-Serag HB. Hepatocellular carcinoma. *N Engl J Med.* 22 Sep 2011; 365: 1118–1127.

European Association for the Study of the Liver. EASL Clinical practice guidelines: Hemochromatosis. Available from http://www.easl.eu/medias/cpg/issue3/Report.pdf.

European Association for the Study of the Liver. EASL clinical practical guidelines: Management of alcoholic liver disease. Available from http://www.easl.eu/medias/cpg/issue9/Report.pdf.

European Association for the Study of the Liver. EASL Clinical practice guidelines: Management of cholestatic liver diseases. Available from http://www.easl.eu/assets/application/files/b664961b2692dc2_file.pdf.

European Association for the Study of the Liver. EASL Clinical practice guidelines: Wilson's disease. Available from http://www.easl.eu/medias/cpg/issue6/Report.pdf.

Farthing M, Salam M, Lindberg, G, *et al*. Acute diarrhea in adults and children: A global perspective. WGO global guidelines. Feb 2012. Available from http://www.worldgastroenterology.org/guidelines/global-guidelines/acute-diarrhea/acute-diarrhea-english.

Fitzgerald RC, di Pietro M, Ragunath K, *et al*. BSG guidelines on the diagnosis and management of Barrett's oesophagus. Available from http://www.bsg.org.uk/images/stories/docs/clinical/guidelines/oesophageal/bsg_barretts_13.pdf.

Forner A, Llovet JM, Bruix J. Hepatocellular carcinoma. *Lancet*. 31 Mar 2012; 379(9822): 1245–1255.

Frossard JL, Steer ML, Pastor CM. Acute pancreatitis. *Lancet*. 12 Jan 2008; 371(9607): 143–152.

Ginès P, Cárdenas A, Arroyo V, Rodés J. Management of cirrhosis and ascites. *N Engl J Med*. 15 Apr 2004; 350(16): 1646–1654.

Ginès P, Guevara M, Arroyo V, Rodés J. Hepatorenal syndrome. *Lancet*. 29 Nov 2003; 362(9398): 1819–1827.

Gleeson D, Heneghan MA. BSG guidelines for management of autoimmune hepatitis. Available from http://www.bsg.org.uk/images/stories/docs/clinical/guidelines/liver/autoimmune_hepatitis_11.pdf.

Gurusamy KS, Davidson BR. Gallstones. *BMJ*. 22 Apr 2014; 348: g2669.

Hartgrink HH, Jensen EP, van Grieken NC, *et al*. Gastric cancer. *Lancet*. 8 Aug 2009; 374(9688): 477–490.

Hidalgo M. Pancreatic cancer. *N Engl J Med*. 15 Jul 2010; 362(17): 1605–1617.

Humes DJ, Simpson J. Acute appendicitis. *BMJ*. 9 Sep 2006; 333(7567): 530–534.

Indar AA, Beckingham IJ. Acute cholecystitis. *BMJ*. 21 Sep 2002; 325(7365): 639–643.

Krawitt EL. Autoimmune hepatitis. *N Engl J Med*. 5 Jan 2006; 354(1): 54–66.

Krige JEJ, Beckingham IJ. Liver abscess and hydatid disease. *BMJ*. 2001; 322.

Lee YM, Kaplan MM. Primary sclerosing cholangitis. *N Engl J Med*. 6 Apr 1995; 332(14): 924–933.

Lucey MR, Mathurin P, Morgan TR. Alcoholic hepatitis. *N Engl J Med*. 25 Jun 2009; 360(26): 2758–2769.

Madoff RD, Parker SC, Varma MG, Lowry AC. Faecal incontinence in adults. *Lancet*. 14 Aug 2004; 364(9434): 621–632.

Maheshwari A, Ray S, Thuluvath PJ. Acute hepatitis C. *Lancet*. 26 Jul 2008; 372(9635) 321–332.

Malfertheiner P, Chan FK, McColl KE. Peptic ulcer disease. *Lancet*. 24 Oct 2009; 374(9699): 1449–1461.

McCallum IJ, Ong S, Mercer-Jones M. Chronic constipation in adults. *BMJ*. 20 Mar 2009; 338: b831.

Mehanna HM, Moledina J, Travis J. Refeeding syndrome: What it is, and how to prevent and treat it. *BMJ*. 28 Jun 2008; 336(7659): 1495–1498.

Menon KV, Shah V, Kamath PS. The Budd-Chiari syndrome. *N Engl J Med*. 5 Feb 2004; 350(6): 578–585.

Miller MH, Agarwal K, Austin A, *et al.* 2014 UK consensus guidelines: Hepatitis C management and direct-acting anti-viral therapy. *Aliment Pharmacol Ther*. 2014; 39(12): 1363–1375.

Modlin IM, Oberg K, Chung DC, *et al.* Gastroenteropancreatic neuroendocrine tumours. *Lancet Oncol*. Jan 2008; 9(1): 61–72.

Moore KP, Aithal GP. Guidelines on the management of ascites in cirrhosis. *Gut*. Oct 2006; 55 Suppl 6: vi1–vi12.

Mowat C, Cole A, Windsor A, *et al.* on behalf of the IBD Section of the British Society of Gastroenterology. Guidelines for the management of inflammatory bowel disease in adults. *Gut*. 2011; 60: 571–607.

Murphy T, Hunt RH, Fried M, Krabshuis JH. World Gastroenterology Organisation practice guidelines: Diverticular disease. 2007. Available from http://www.worldgastroenterology.org/UserFiles/file/guidelines/diverticular-disease-english-2007.pdf.

National Institute for Health and Care Excellence. Acute upper gastrointestinal bleeding in over 16s: Management. NICE guidelines [CG141]. June 2012. Available from http://www.nice.org.uk/guidance/CG141.

National Institute for Health and Care Excellence. Colorectal cancer: Diagnosis and management. NICE guidelines [CG131]. Nov 2011. Available from https://www.nice.org.uk/guidance/cg131.

National Institute for Health and Care Excellence. Gastro-oesophageal reflux disease and dyspepsia in adults: Investigation and management. NICE guidelines [CG184]. Sep 2014. Available from https://www.nice.org.uk/guidance/cg184.

National Institute for Health and Care Excellence. Hepatitis B (chronic): Diagnosis and management. NICE guidelines [CG165]. June 2013. Available from https://www.nice.org.uk/Guidance/CG165.

National Institute for Health and Care Excellence. Nutrition support for adults: Oral nutrition support, enteral tube feeding and parenteral nutrition. NICE guidelines [CG32]. Feb 2006. Available from http://www.nice.org.uk/guidance/cg32.

Pancreatic Section of the British Society of Gastroenterology, Pancreatic Society of Great Britain and Ireland, Association of Upper Gastrointestinal Surgeons of Great Britain and Ireland, Royal College of Pathologists, Special Interest Group for Gastro-I. Guidelines for the management of patients with pancreatic cancer periampullary and ampullary carcinomas. *Gut.* Jun 2005; 54 Suppl 5: v1–16.

Paterson WG, Goyal RK, Habib FI. Esophageal motility disorders. *GI Motility Online.* 2006. doi:10.1038/gimo20.

Pennathur A, Gibson MK, Jobe BA, Luketich JD. Oesophageal carcinoma. *Lancet.* 2 Feb 2013; 381(9864): 400–412.

Ramage JK, Ahmed A, Ardill J, *et al.* UK and Ireland Neuroendocrine Tumour Society. Guidelines for the management of gastroenteropancreatic neuroendocrine (including carcinoid) tumours (NETs). *Gut.* Jan 2012; 61(1): 6–32.

Ratnaike R. Whipple's disease. *Postgrad Med J.* Dec 2000; 76(902): 760–766.

Roberts EA, Schilsky ML. Diagnosis and treatment of Wilson disease: An update. AASLD practice guidelines. Available from https://www.aasld.org/sites/default/files/guideline_documents/Wilson%20Disease2009.pdf.

Roman S, Kahrilas PJ. The diagnosis and management of hiatus hernia. *BMJ.* 23 Oct 2014; 349: g6154.

Ryder SD, Beckingham IJ. Acute hepatitis. *BMJ.* 2001; 322.

Scottish Intercollegiate Guidelines Network. Management of acute upper and lower gastrointestinal bleeding. Sep 2008. Available from http://www.sign.ac.uk/pdf/sign105.pdf.

Selmi C, Bowlus CL, Gershwin ME, Coppel RL. Primary biliary cirrhosis. *Lancet.* 7 May 2011; 377(9777):1600 –1609.

Shaheen NJ, Richter JE. Barrett's oesophagus. *Lancet.* 7–13 March 2009; 373(9666): 850–861.

Silverman EK, Sandhaus RA. Clinical practice: Alpha 1 antitrypsin deficiency. *N Engl J Med.* 25 Jun 2009; 360(26): 2749–2757.

Spiller R, Aziz Q, Creed F, *et al*. Guidelines on the irritable bowel syndrome: Mechanisms and practical management. *Gut*. 2007; 56(12): 1770–1798.

Sreenarasimhaiah J. Diagnosis and management of intestinal ischaemic disorders. *BMJ*. 21 Jun 2003; 326(7403): 1372–1376.

Srirajaskanthan R, Shanmugabavan D, Ramage JK. Carcinoid syndrome. *BMJ*. 23 Aug 2010; 341: c3941.

Stoller JK, Aboussouan LS. Alpha 1-antitrypsin deficiency. *Lancet*. 25 Jun 2005; 365(9478): 2225–2236.

Thomas PD, Forbes A, Green J, *et al*. Guidelines for the investigation of chronic diarrhoea, 2nd edition. *Gut*. Jul 2003; 52 Suppl 5: v1–v15.

Trépo C, Chan HL, Lok A. Hepatitis B virus infection. *Lancet*. 6 Dec 2014; 384(9959): 2053–2063.

Tsochatzis, EA, Bosch J, Burroughs AK. Liver cirrhosis. *Lancet*. 17 May 2014; 383(9930): 1749–1761.

Vasen HF, Blanco I, Aktan-Collan K, *et al*. Mallorca group. Revised guidelines for the clinical management of Lynch syndrome (HNPCC): Recommendations by a group of European experts. *Gut*. Jun 2013; 62(6): 812–823.

Vasen HF, Möslein G, Alonso A, *et al*. Guidelines for the clinical management of familial adenomatous polyposis (FAP). *Gut*. May 2008; 57(5): 704–713.

Williams EJ, Green J, Beckingham I, *et al*.; British Society of Gastroenterology. Guidelines on the management of common bile duct stones (CBDS). *Gut*. Jul 2008; 57(7): 1004–1021.

Working party of the British Society of Gastroenterology; Association of Surgeons of Great Britain and Ireland; Pancreatic Society of Great Britain and Ireland; Association of Upper Gastrointestinal Surgeons of Great Britain and Ireland. UK guidelines for the management of acute pancreatitis. *Gut*. May 2005; 54 Suppl 3: iii1–9.

Disclaimer

This text was produced in reference to current guidelines. At the time of publication there may have been further updates to the evidence and the reader is advised to be aware of this fact. Furthermore any drugs listed may or may not have drug dosages listed to minimise potential errors. Readers are advised to refer to the latest pharmaceutical formularies for clarification.

Notes

Part II

Cardiology

Heart Failure (Chronic)

Aetiopathogenesis

Chronic heart failure is associated with significant remodelling. Evidence suggests the occurrence of cardiomyocyte hypertrophy with alterations in calcium handling and contractile abilities. There also exists remodelling of the extracellular matrix with fibrosis and matrix metalloproteinase activation. The hypertrophic pathway is significantly complex and a detailed understanding is not required. However elements of interest involved include insulin like growth factor, Phosphoinositide 3-kinase alpha and protein kinase B in relation to physiological remodelling. Pathological remodelling focuses on activation of G protein coupled receptors, tyrosine kinase receptors and natriuretic peptide receptors. The remodelling process also centres on microRNAs (miRs) which are implicated in myocyte hypertrophy, fibrosis, excitation contraction, dilatation and apoptosis.

Failing myocytes are associated with a decrease in calcium amplitude and raised diastolic calcium concentration with increased calcium leakage. Along with apoptosis, there is also autophagy, a self-digesting recycling process. Fibrosis is typically due to TGF β involvement and fibroblast activation.

Hormonal influences also exist in the development of heart failure. This occurs due to a reduction in cardiac output leading to production of adrenaline, noradrenaline and activation of the renin angiotensin system. Vasoconstriction occurs with aldosterone release and retention of salt as well as water further straining the cardiac system. Overtime the counterbalancing vasodilatory system, via nitric oxide, prostaglandins, Atrial natriuretic peptide and Brain natriuretic peptide fails.

165

Numerous causes of heart failure exist. These include coronary artery disease, diabetes, hypertension, valvular dysfunction, pulmonary disease such as a PE, infections, drugs (alcohol, cocaine, doxorubicin), cardiomyopathies, anaemia, hyperthyroidism and B1 deficiency.

Symptoms

Dyspnoea on exertion
Orthopnoea
Dyspnoea at rest
Paroxysmal nocturnal dyspnoea
Chest pain
Palpitations
Fatigue
Weakness

Confusion and headaches (note in case of cerebrovascular atherosclerosis, often forgotten)

The New York Heart Association is a well-recognised strategy for symptom classification in relation to heart failure

I.   No limitation of physical activity. Ordinary physical activity does not cause undue fatigue, palpitations, dyspnoea (shortness of breath).

II. Slight limitation of physical activity. Comfortable at rest. Ordinary physical activity results in fatigue, palpitations, dyspnoea (shortness of breath).

III. Marked limitation of physical activity. Comfortable at rest. Less than ordinary activity causes fatigue, palpitations, or dyspnoea.

IV. Unable to carry on any physical activity without discomfort. Symptoms of heart failure at rest. If any physical activity is undertaken, discomfort increases.

Signs

Elevated JVP

Central/ peripheral cyanosis

Malar flush

Diminished pulse pressure

Ascites secondary to increased hepatic vein pressures

Hepatomegaly

Evidence of pulmonary oedema/ peripheral oedema

Tricuspid and mitral regurgitation

S3 gallop due to rapid ventricular filling

Pulsus alternans secondary to impaired LV ejection

Enhanced P2 in view of increased pulmonary artery pressures

Differentials

Acute respiratory distress syndrome

Pneumonia

COPD

Pulmonary fibrosis

PE

Nephrotic syndrome

Pulmonary oedema

Investigations

A primary investigation of choice is transthoracic 2D echocardiography as well as measurement of serum BNP or N-terminalproBNP. An urgent referral for an ECHO is typically based on a BNP above 400 pg/ml or an NTproBNP > 2000 pg/ml. Note that high levels of serum natriuretic peptides can also be seen in conditions such as renal failure, sepsis, COPD and diabetes. A transoesophageal ECHO is of merit in cases where imaging from a transthoracic echocardiogram has been minimalistic say for example in those who are massively obese or are mechanically ventilated. Additional imaging of choice may be a cardiac CT or MRI. Radionuclide imaging can be useful assessment wise focusing on ventricular function and wall motion.

Additional investigations include a full blood count (assessing for evidence of anaemia or infection), renal function assessment, liver function measurement, fasting lipids, glucose, thyroid function tests and urinalysis to assess for the presence of proteinuria along with peak flow and spirometry. A chest X ray helps to ascertain the presence of pulmonary oedema. And of course do not forget the need for an ECG which will help to indicate the presence of arrhythmias or ischaemia. Note the presence for example of left bundle branch block or left ventricular hypertrophy. Arterial blood gas measurement although not routinely performed in heart failure helps to ascertain the degree of hypoxia or hypercapnia and hence severity of pathology. If one suspects coronary artery disease as the possible cause then coronary angiography is essential.

Management

Initial recommendations include a focus on lifestyle factors such as exercise, stopping smoking if applicable and abstaining from alcohol. If there is evidence of left ventricular dysfunction consider an ACE inhibitor and β Blocker. If symptoms remain despite such medication the next advisable treatment regimen would be an aldosterone antagonist or an angiotensin II receptor antagonist. Hydralazine along with a nitrate is advisable for those who are African or Caribbean who also have moderate to severe heart impairment. Points to note include the fact that patients on ACE inhibitors should have an assessment of their renal function with inclusion of eGFR at the commencement and following each dose increase. β blockers require an assessment of heart rate and blood pressure during each dose change.

Aldosterone antagonists also require renal function monitoring paying close attention to serum potassium levels. An angiotensin II receptor blocker as highlighted earlier is typically instigated in those who are unable to tolerate the side effects of an ACE inhibitor.

Digoxin is an option for those with continued worsening heart failure whereby treatment options as highlighted above fail to provide benefit. Diuretic agents such as furosemide as a loop diuretic is an advantageous agent for the relief of fluid retention. Calcium channel blockers are also useful such as amlodipine. Appropriate liver and thyroid function monitoring is advisable. Consider anticoagulant usage in those with co-existing thromboembolic disease and inotropic agents such as dobutamine in the acute relapse of chronic heart failure. Severe heart failure which remains refractory to medical treatment requires cardiac transplantation. It is important to note that all chronic heart failure patients should be offered tailored exercise based rehabilitation.

Implantable cardioverter defibrillator and cardiac resynchronisation therapy is a recommended therapeutic intervention in patients with heart failure who have evidence of left ventricular dysfunction and a left ventricular ejection fraction < 35%.

A Note on Acute Heart Failure

Management

Intravenous diuretic therapy is essential in the acute management of heart failure. Inotropes or vasopressors in acute heart failure should be provided in those with potential evidence of reversible cardiogenic shock. It is advisable that such treatment occurs in a high dependency setting as a minimum. If there is evidence of cardiogenic pulmonary oedema in addition to dyspnoea and acidaemia, non-invasive ventilation is advisable. Surgical intervention is employed where valvular dysfunction has been responsible for resulting heart failure. Furthermore patients may benefit from mechanical assist devices if there is evidence of reversible severe acute heart failure or for patients with the potential benefit for transplantation.

Acute Coronary Syndrome

Aetiopathogenesis

The primary trigger for acute coronary syndrome is fissuring or rupture of an atheromatous plaque in the coronary artery. The end result
is a thrombotic response leading to blood flow obstruction and resulting
ischaemic damage. Various factors can enhance the risk of ACS including
increasing age, male gender, positive family history, smoking, diabetes,
hypertension, obesity, psychosocial factors, excess alcohol consumption
and poor diet lacking fruits and vegetables.

Symptoms

Chest pain which can radiate (neck, shoulder, back)
Sweating
Shortness of breath
Palpitations
Nausea

Typically symptoms are worsened by exertion and relieved by rest. However this is not always the case.

Signs

Hypotension/ hypertension
Evidence of heart failure as previously described

Differentials

Asthma
Oesophagitis

Pericarditis

Cardiomyopathy

MI

Myocarditis

Investigations

A 12 lead ECG is the paramount investigation of choice which should be repeated regularly if concerns remain regarding the diagnostic picture. Typical findings include T and ST segment changes/left bundle branch block. Serum troponin measurement is essential at presentation and three hours post.

Additional investigations include a chest X ray, ECHO, myocardial perfusion assessment, cardiac angiography/CT coronary angiography.

Management

Patients with acute coronary syndrome with evidence of ischaemic ECG changes and cardiac troponin enzyme elevation should receive treatment with both aspirin (300 mg loading) and ticagrelor (180 mg loading). For those individuals undergoing PCI aspirin and prasugrel (60 mg loading) can be instigated.

If the risk of bleeding is presumed greater than the benefits of reducing further cardiac thrombotic events then the most suitable option is the use of aspirin and clopidogrel (300 mg loading) as opposed to ticagrelor or prasugrel.

It is important to note that in the existence of ischaemic ECG changes or elevated cardiac enzymes the treatment of choice is fondaparinux/ low molecular weight heparin. ST segment elevation ACS patients will also benefit from fondaparinux who do not receive reperfusion intervention.

β blockers should be commenced where significant hypotension or bradycardia does not exist. Those patients with diabetes mellitus/ significant hyperglycaemia require glucose monitoring and an insulin glucose infusion.

ST segment events require immediate primary Percutaneous Coronary Intervention. And in house guidelines are available for transfer to proximity interventional centres. This is typically stent based. If PCI can not be provided within 120 minutes then immediate thrombolysis is advised with agents such as Tissue plasminogen activator/alteplase. ST segment elevation acute coronary syndrome within 6 hours of symptom commencement who fail to reperfuse require rescue PCI.

Risk stratification is an element of importance and is based on Global Registry of Acute Coronary Events utilisation.

Age (years)		ST-segment deviation	☐
Heart rate (bpm)		Cardiac arrest at admission	☐
Systolic blood pressure (mmHg)		Elevated troponin*	☐
CHF (Killip class)		* Or other necrosis cardiac biomarkers	
Diuretic usage	☐		
Creatinine (mg dL $^{-1}$/mmol L $^{-1}$)			
Renal failure	☐		

The Killip classification:

   I. No clinical sign of CHF
  II. Presence of rales (crackles) in the lungs, raised jugular venous pressure, or third heart sound (S3 gallop)
 III. Acute pulmonary oedema
  IV. Cardiogenic shock

In addition, non ST segment elevation patients at risk of recurrent events should receive angiography and revascularisation. ST segment ACS patients who have undergone thrombolytic therapy should receive coronary angiography and revascularisation. Glycoprotein IIb/IIIa receptor blockers should be offered at the time of PCI where adverse risk may be a concern. For non ST segment elevation ACS, coronary artery bypass graft is often implemented for those with diabetes mellitus, left main stem disease or multi vessel disease.

Long term aspirin at 75 mg is advised for patients. And 6 months of dual anti platelet intervention is advised along with statin therapy and β blockade. Myocardial ischaemia related chest pain benefits from nitrates. Unstable angina occurrence requires long term ACE inhibitors as does a MI. Intolerance to ACE inhibitors relies on ARBs in the presence of left ventricular dysfunction/ heart failure. Heart failure and diabetic patients with a MI impaired by left ventricular impairment, namely an ejection fraction < 40%, rely on eplerenone.

Cardiac surgical intervention should be undertaken in view of possible mechanical complications of an acute MI such as wall or muscle rupture.

At this point it is worth highlighting the management of stable angina

Stable Angina

Management

Management of choice relies on the use of short acting nitrates. Side effects include flushing and headaches as well as light headiness. When a short acting nitrate is being utilised repeated doses are beneficial if the pain remains. 75 mg aspirin is advisable along with ACE inhibitors and statins. Further agents of value include β blockers and calcium channel blockers. If such agents are contra indicated then revert to nitrate therapy, ivabradine, nicorandil or ranolazine.

If medical therapy fails to improve symptomatology the next option relies on CABG or PCI intervention.

A Note on Cardiogenic Shock

Management

If the occurrence of cardiogenic shock occurs secondary to a MI the first choice of treatment is PCI or CABG if PCI is not suitable.

Fluid support is essential typically 250-500 ml of crystalloid with vasopressor use such as noradrenaline. A mean arterial pressure of 65–75 mmHg is advisable. Inotropes should also be employed if tissue hypoperfusion remains following fluid use and MAP optimisation. Examples include dobutamine and milrinone.

Mechanical cardiac based support is needed when the above strategies fail to evoke improvement in both tissue and oxygen perfusion and the risk of multi organ failure enhances. The intra-aortic balloon pump device helps to improve coronary blood flow, reduce left ventricular afterload/ myocardial oxygen consumption and pulmonary capillary wedge pressure with an increase in cardiac output.

Left ventricular assist devices are more beneficial than IABPs but are more invasive. Extracorporeal membrane oxygenation is the next stage for total circulatory support.

Monitoring of patients in cardiogenic shock relies on the use of pulmonary artery catheterization (PAC) for those patients who are haemodynamically unstable with evidence of hypoperfusion. PAC provides data on pulmonary arterial and cardiac filling pressures, mixed venous saturation and thermodilution derived cardiac output.

Hypertension

Aetiopathogenesis

Hypertension can be deemed primary or secondary to a specific cause. Genetic influences have highlighted the occurrence of mutations that can impede the functioning of the sodium chloride co transporter and potassium channels. In essential hypertension one observes a progression from increased cardiac output secondary to sodium renal retention. Following this there is hyper adrenergic activity with later developments focusing on vascular remodelling and subsequent vaso constriction.

Causes of hypertension are numerous and may include renal based pathology such as polycystic kidney disease, glomerulonephritis, renal malignancy leading to excess renin production or Liddle syndrome. Renovascular hypertension is also worthy of interest occurring secondary to vascular issues such as collagen vascular dysfunction, vasculitis or aortic coarctation. Various endocrine causes exist such as Cushing's syndrome, primary hyper aldosteronism, phaeochromocytoma, acromegaly, diabetes, hyperparathyroidism and Congenital adrenal hyperplasia. Other aetiologies include central nervous system dysfunction, obesity, drugs such as alcohol, cocaine, nonsteroidal anti-inflammatory drugs, the oral contraceptive pill and steroids.

Symptoms

Chest pain
Symptoms associated with heart failure
Headache
Dizziness

Blurred vision

Nausea/ vomiting

Symptoms allied to underlying cause

It is important to note however that patients with an elevated blood pressure often do not have symptoms.

Signs

Hypertensive retinopathy

Absent or delayed pulses

Renal artery bruits

Left ventricular hypertrophy (displaced apex beat, S4)

Differentials

Heart failure

Stroke

Cardiomyopathy

MI

Hyperthyroidism

Investigations

Measurement of blood pressure is fundamental of course. Repeated measurements are advised and on both arms. If repeated measurements remain greater than 140/ 90 mm Hg ambulatory measurements are required.

Further investigations help to determine a possible cause. These include blood glucose measurements, renal function, lipid profile and thyroid function tests as well as urine screening for protein and blood. Consider CT angiography for aortic coarctation, 24 hour measurement of urinary metanephrine/ normetanephrine for phaeochromocytoma, aldosterone: renin ratio measurements for primary aldosteronism, Doppler flow and angiography for reno vascular hypertension and additional tests as necessary to exclude the underlying cause.

Management

Current guidelines trichotomise hypertension as follows:

Stage 1 — > 140/ 90 mm Hg,
Stage 2 — > 160/ 100 mm Hg,
Severe — > 180/ 110 mm Hg.

Lifestyle intervention is valuable with a focus on smoking, alcohol, diet and exercise. Caffeine and sodium intake should be reduced.

Initial treatment of choice for those aged < 55 years includes an ACE inhibitor or Angiotensin receptor blocker. Patients over the age of 55 and black or Afro Caribbean individuals require a calcium channel blocker or a thiazide diuretic agent. Preferred agents include chlortalidone or indapamide. β blockers are not preferred agents generally in the management of hypertension but come into play in view of contraindications to ACE inhibitors or ARBs or in women of child bearing age.

If blood pressure control remains an issue despite the above regimens one can utilise a combination of a calcium channel blocker with an ACE inhibitor or ARB. Thiazide diuretics are of course substituted for a calcium channel blocker if not suitable say in the case of oedema or intolerance. Black or Afro Caribbean individuals benefit from ARB agents along with calcium channel blockers.

Persistent hypertension then requires spironolactone with careful monitoring of serum potassium. Additional agents of interest at this point include an alpha or β blocker.

What is particularly of importance in the management of hypertension is the need for regular dosing and compliance assessments.

Infective Endocarditis (IE)

Aetiopathogenesis

The primary trigger for infective endocarditis is initial endothelial injury leading to the release of cytokines and tissue factors resulting in thrombus formation and subsequent bacterial adherence which leads overtime to bacterial mass clumping. Initial endothelial damage occurs as a result of valve sclerosis or bacterial influence itself. The most common bacterial triggers include Staphylococcus, Streptococcus and Enterococcus.

It is important to have a broad overview of the primary factors that are responsible for IE. Factors may include rheumatic valve disease, valve prolapse, congenital heart disease, prosthetic valve disease, IV drug misuse, therapeutic interventions such as line insertion and pacemakers.

Symptoms

Fever
Shortness of breath
Cough
Joint pain
Headaches
Myalgia
Symptoms indicative of heart failure

Signs

Splinter haemorrhages
Petechiae
Osler's nodes

Janeway lesions

Roth spots

Note any evidence of neurological dysfunction or bone/ joint dysfunction pain in view of embolic occurrences

Splenomegaly (embolic related)

Differentials

Atrial myxoma

Polymyalgia Rheumatica

Reactive arthritis

Systemic lupus erythematosus

Investigations

Initial blood investigations are focused on a full blood count and C-reactive protein assessment for evidence of infection in addition to an erythrocyte sedimentation rate. Urine screens may reveal evidence of proteinuria and haematuria secondary to renal infarction. Further investigations may include a pro calcitonin level but typically this is nonspecific. Imaging is typically a transthoracic ECHO in the first instance. However if there is still strong suspicion of IE then a transesophageal echocardiogram is advised. If both the TTE and TOE are negative yet suspicion remains high of IE, then these investigations should be repeated within at least a 7 day time frame. A TOE is advised in those patients with evidence of a prosthetic heart valve or intracardiac device.

Blood cultures are advisable in those patients ideally before commencing treatment. Guidelines have advised appropriate aseptic technique and a minimum of three sets peripherally with a greater than 6 hour interval before antimicrobial treatment has been started. The Duke criteria, below, is designed to aid in the diagnosis of IE.

Pathological criteria: Microorganisms on histology or culture of a vegetation or intracardiac abscess Evidence of lesions: vegetation or intracardiac abscess showing active endocarditis on histology

Major clinical criteria 1) Blood cultures positive for infective endocarditis Typical microorganisms consistent with infective endocarditis from two separate blood cultures: • Staphylococcus aureus, Viridans streptococci, Streptococcus bovis, HACEK (Haemophilus, Aggregatibacter, Cardio-bacterium, Eikenella corrodens, Kingella) group, or community-acquired enterococci, in the absence of a primary focus or microorganisms consistent with infective endocarditis from persistently positive blood cultures: • At least two positive blood cultures from blood samples drawn >12 h apart, or • All of three, or most of ≥4 separate cultures of blood (with first and last sample >1 h apart) or Single positive blood culture for Coxiella burnetii, or phase 1 IgG antibody titre >1:800 2) Evidence of endocardial involvement Echocardiography positive for infective endocarditis • Defined by presence of a vegetation, abscess, or new partial dehiscence of prosthetic valve New valvular regurgitation • Note—increase or change in pre-existing murmur is not sufficient

Minor clinical criteria 1) Predisposition: predisposing heart condition, intravenous drug use 2) Fever: temperature >38°C 3) Vascular phenomena: major arterial emboli, septic pulmonary infarcts, mycotic aneurysm, intracranial haemorrhages, conjunctival haemorrhages, Janeway lesions 4) Immunological phenomena: glomerulonephritis, Osler's nodes, Roth spots, rheumatoid factor 5) Microbiological evidence: positive blood culture that does not meet a major criterion or serological evidence of active infection with organism consistent with infective endocarditis. Diagnosis of infective endocarditis is definite in the presence of one pathological criterion, or two major criteria, or one major and three minor criteria, or five minor criteria. Diagnosis of infective endocarditis is possible in the presence of one major and one minor criteria, or three minor criteria

Those patients with a suspicion of IE with significant sepsis should undergo two sets of blood cultures within one hour. Further advice focuses on the need of serology for Coxiella and Bartonella in individuals with negative blood culture infective endocarditis.

Surgical intervention should be prompted in patients with prosthetic intracardiac endocarditis.

Management

The recommended empirical treatment regimens for IE are as follows:

Native valve endocarditis benefits from amoxicillin and gentamicin. If there is evidence of severe sepsis then patients should undergo the combination regimen of vancomycin and gentamicin. If there is evidence of risk factors for Pseudomonas / Enterobacteriaceae, vancomycin and meropenem are worthy agents of choice. Prosthetic valves benefit from vancomycin, gentamicin and rifampicin. It is important to note that the dosing and levels of agents such as gentamicin and vancomycin need guidance from in house pharmacists. In cases of renal failure, dosing of gentamicin needs adjusting accordingly. Ciprofloxacin is preferred as opposed to gentamicin if concerns exist in terms of nephrotoxicity. Some organisms of choice that should be considered are as follows:

Staphylococcal — flucloxacillin. For MRSA or those with a penicillin
    allergy recommendations include vancomycin plus rifampicin. Dap-
    tomycin is an alternative for those intolerant of vancomycin
Streptococcal — benzylpenicillin/ ceftriaxone/ gentamicin
HACEK — cephalosporin/ amoxicillin with initial gentamicin addition
Enterococcal — amoxicillin with gentamicin
Fungal — fluconazole, variconazole, amphotericin B

Surgical intervention in IE is advised for those patients with resultant heart failure, continuing uncontrolled infection with fever persistence, abscess and vegetations. It is important to note that vegetations typically greater than 10 mm pose an embolic threat hence the surgical need.

Pericardial Diseases

Aetiopathogenesis

Numerous causes exist for the occurrence of pericarditis. These include infectious causes such as viruses (eg Coxsackie, Mumps, Epstein Barr virus, Cytomegalovirus, Varicella, Rubella, HIV, Parvovirus B19), bacterial (e.g meningococcal, pneumococcal, haemophilus, chlamydia, TB) and fungal. Autoimmune diseases are also accountable such as systemic lupus erythematosus and rheumatoid arthritis. Additional pathology may contribute to disease such as metabolic disorders (diabetes, uraemia, Addison's, hypothyroidism) pregnancy and malignancy. Constrictive pericarditis occurs commonly due to TB, mediastinal irradiation and previous cardiac surgery. Cardiac tamponade occurs typically due to drugs such as cyclosporine and anticoagulants, cardiac surgery, trauma, connective tissue disease, renal failure and malignancy.

Symptoms

In view of the array of diseases in this section bullet points have been avoided. Acute pericarditis (AP) is typically associated with chest pain, fever and malaise. The pain can be pleuritic and alters with posture. Chronic pericarditis is linked with milder symptoms, namely chest pain, palpitations and fatigue. Constrictive pericarditis is linked with fatigue and dyspnoea.

Signs

AP can be associated with a pericardial friction rub and pleural effusion. Constrictive pericarditis may be associated with oedema and abdominal distension as well as muscle wasting secondary to a protein losing enteropathy. It is also usually associated with Kussmaul's sign and a peri-cardial knock. Cardiac tamponade presents with an elevated JVP, hypo-tension, pulsus paradoxus and tachypnoea.

Differentials

The list of differentials are extensive. Examples include:

Angina

Aortic dissection

Oesophageal rupture

GORD

MI

Peptic ulcer disease

PE

Investigations

In regards to acute pericarditis, an ECG will demonstrate anterior/inferior concave ST segment elevation and PR segment deviations pro-gressing to T wave flattening. An ECHO helps to determine the pres-ence/absence of an effusion. Blood investigations are focused on inflam-matory marker use namely the ESR, CRP and lactate dehydrogenase with request for a troponin as a marker for myocardial damage. Further imaging may rely on a chest X ray, CT or MRI. A pericardial biopsy with fluid analysis can help to determine the aetiology in question.

In the case of cardiac tamponade one observes ST/T wave changes, electrical alternans or electromechanical dissociation. An ECHO will indicate diastolic collapse of the atria/ventricles with cardiac catheter-isation highlighting elevated right atrial pressures, pulmonary artery diastolic pressures and pulmonary capillary wedge pressures. For con-strictive pericarditis, an ECG may highlight T wave inversion, low QRS voltage or AV block. A chest X ray will highlight calcification with an ECHO indicating pericardial thickening and calcification along with atrial enlargement. Further imaging such as a CT/MRI may be useful which may demonstrate a thickened pericardium. An endomyocardial biopsy is often non specific with possible myocyte hypertrophy/ myocardial fibrosis.

Management

The treatment of acute pericarditis relies on the use of nonsteroidal anti-inflammatory drugs. Ibuprofen is a good agent of choice with appropriate gastro intestinal protection. Colchicine may also prove useful as well as steroids. Chronic pericarditis also follows the same treatment regimen. Both acute and chronic pericarditis may require pericardiocentesis if there exists an effusion > 20 mm on ECHO imaging during diastole. Contraindications to pericardiocentesis are aortic dissection, coagulation disorders and thrombocytopenia. A pericardiectomy may prove beneficial in chronic pericarditis. In cases of recurrent pericarditis, medical treatments comprising colchicine, NSAIDS and steroids are worthwhile. Alternatives to steroids include azathioprine, or cyclophosphamide. And again an impaired response to medication will benefit from a pericardiectomy. If in the case of constrictive pericarditis, the optimum treatment of choice is pericardiectomy. It is important to emphasise the importance of treating the underlying cause in all cases.

Hypertrophic Obstructive Cardio-myopathy (HOCM)

Aetiopathogenesis

Typically HOCM is genetic based with sarcomeric protein gene mutations inherited in an autosomal dominant fashion. Mutations may be missense or truncating observed in genes encoding myosin heavy chain, cardiac muscle β isoform (MYH7), cardiac myosin binding protein C or cardiac muscle troponin T. Non sarcomere genetic involvements have been recognised including GLA, TTR and LAMP 2.

Non genetic causes are of importance and comprise drugs such as steroids or tacrolimus and amyloidosis.

In HOCM, one observes intraventricular obstruction at the left ventricular outflow tract but also at the midventricular element. Left ventricular obstruction is secondary to systolic anterior motion of the mitral apparatus towards the hypertrophied septum. Mid ventricular obstruction is secondary to hypertrophied papillary muscles and mid ventricular hypertrophy. Currently, it is not fully clear why sarcomeric mutations result in pathology. Evidence suggests that such mutations lead to a hypercontractile state secondary to an increase in ATPase activity, calcium sensitivity and increased sarcomere force production. Additional factors of interest include excess production of catecholamines, thickened coronary arteries and cardiac anatomical impairment.

Symptoms

Shortness of breath
Chest pain
Palpitations

Syncope

Dizziness

Orthopnoea

Signs

Double/ triple apical impulse

Double carotid arterial pulse

Split S2

S4

Ejection systolic murmur between apex and left of sternum radiating to sternal notch

Mitral regurgitation

Differentials

Restrictive cardiomyopathy

Heart failure

Aortic stenosis

Investigations

Investigations of choice include an ECG which can demonstrate P wave abnormalities, Q waves, left axis deviation and inverted T waves. A 2D ECHO is needed to help confirm evidence of hypertrophy, namely a wall thickness of 15 mm or more and systolic anterior motion of the mitral apparatus.

Cardiac MRI will detect interstitial fibrosis with evidence of late gadolinium enhancement. Further imaging relies on Positron Emission Tomography scanning to help ascertain evidence of ischaemia. Exercise stress testing should also be employed primarily as a risk stratification tool as well as genetic testing.

Management

The primary treatment of choice is β Blockers or verapamil. However verapamil should not be used in those with marked obstruction or elevated pulmonary arterial pressures. If these agents fail to provide benefit, disopyramide or cibenzoline should be used. To alleviate any existence of congestive based symptoms, diuretic therapy is of advantage.

If symptoms remain despite medical therapy then patients should undergo septal reduction therapy with reduction of left ventricular outflow tract obstruction achieved following approximately 5-10 g of myocardial removal from the basal interventricular septum. Additional interventions include resection of the myocardium in the middle or apical segment of the interventricular septum, plication of mitral valve leaflets, removal of thickened secondary chordae or reorientation of papillary muscles.

An alternative to surgical myectomy is alcoholic ablation. Alternatives to septal reduction include AV pacing. Associated heart failure symptoms should be treated with a compliment of ACE inhibitors, diuretics and mineralocorticoid receptor antagonists. Due to the risk of sudden cardiac death in patients with HOCM, recommendations include the use of an implantable cardioverter-defibrillator.

Dilated Cardiomyopathy

Aetiopathogenesis

Numerous causes exist for the occurrence of dilated cardiomyopathy (DCM). Causes of common interest include cardiac disease such as ischaemia or hypertension, infection eg viral (coxsackie, HIV, CMV, hepatitis, Respiratory syncytial virus, influenza)/ bacterial, endocrine dysfunction, rheumatological disease (SLE/ RA), malnutrition, neurological conditions such as myotonic dystrophy and drugs such as chemotherapeutic agents. DCM can also be of idiopathic occurrence, with the diagnostic criteria highlighted below.

Strong genetic factors exist and include cardiac troponin T, cardiac actin, desmoplakin and dystrophin to name but a few. Inheritance modes encompass autosomal dominance, recessive and X linked. Overall the primary pathophysiological elements in reference to DCM centre on defective force generation and force transmission.

Criteria

- Ejection fraction <0.45 and/or a fractional shortening of <25%
- Left ventricle end diastolic diameter of >117%

Exclusion criteria

- Absence of systemic hypertension (>160/100 mmHg)
- Coronary artery disease (50% in one or more branches)
- Chronic excess alcohol (>40 g/day female, >80 g/day for male)
- Systemic disease known to cause idiopathic dilated cardiomyopathy
- Pericardial disease

- Congenital heart disease
- Cor pulmonale

Symptoms
Fatigue
Shortness of breath
Orthopnoea

Signs
Hyper or hypotension
Cyanosis
Clubbing
Evidence of pulmonary oedema (crepitations for example)
S3
Elevated JVP
Displaced apex beat
Palpable heaves

Differentials
ACS
Pericarditis
Cardiac tamponade
Hypertrophic cardiomyopathy
Restrictive cardiomyopathy
Myocarditis

Investigations
An ECHO will demonstrate evidence of left ventricular dilation and impaired systolic function, namely a worsening ejection fraction. There may be associated evidence of mitral regurgitation and pericardial effusion presence. A chest X ray can help to determine the presence of cardiomegaly with pulmonary oedema. An ECG may show

evidence of sinus tachycardia with ST changes, bundle branch block and left ventricular hypertrophy. Biomarker measurement is necessary namely brain natriuretic peptide and N terminal BNP. Cardiac biopsy sampling can help to determine disease cause. For example viral myocarditis may be ascertained from histology. Further analysis may demonstrate fibrosis/ necrosis and cellular infiltrates.

Management

The management of dilated cardiomyopathy focuses on the allied symptoms of heart failure. The detailed treatment of heart failure has been discussed elsewhere. Therapies of value include ACE inhibitors, β blockers and diuretic intervention. Vasodilators also prove worthwhile such as nitrogylcerin. Assist devices then come into play if medical therapy fails to provide benefit. ICD devices are recommended as well as cardiac resynchronisation therapy.

Surgical management in the form of cardiac transplantation is the final interventional stage typically for patients on inotropes along with ventilator and device based support already in hand.

Restrictive Cardiomyopathy

Aetiopathogenesis

Numerous causes exist for the development of restrictive cardiomyopathy. These may be non infiltrative such as diabetes related or infiltrative, namely amyloidosis, sarcoidosis or fatty infiltration. Storage disease is also a common factor such as haemochromatosis and glycogen storage disease. Additional causes include endomyocardial fibrosis, hypereosinophilic syndrome, radiation, metastatic cancers, carcinoid and drugs such as serotonin and anthracyclines.

One observes from a pathophysiological perspective, increased stiffness of the myocardium, increasing pressure build up in the ventricles with resulting diastolic heart failure.

Symptoms

Shortness of breath
Fatigue
Chest pain
Syncope

Signs

Prominent apical impulse
S3
Regurgitant murmurs
Kussmaul's sign may be present

Differentials

Pericarditis

Cardiac tamponade

Constrictive pericarditis

HOCM

Investigations

An ECG can demonstrate an array of findings. These include low voltage, left axis deviation, AF and conduction defects. An ECHO may demonstrate increased wall thickness and evidence of an underlying cause (eg granular sparkling texture in the case of amyloid). The underlying cause can also be determined from an endomyocardial biopsy. Doppler studies are further investigation tools of value demonstrating reduced right ventricular and left ventricular velocities. CT/ MRI imaging will indicate no pericardial thickening. Cardiac catheterization may highlight a left ventricular end-diastolic pressure > 5 mm Hg higher than the RVEDP.

Management

Symptomatic relief is key with the use of beta blockers/calcium channel blockers and low dose diuretics. If amyloidosis is the underlying cause treatment with melphalan may provide benefit. Venesection and iron chelation therapy is of use in haemochromatosis. Conduction dysfunction is best treated with a pacemaker. A last treatment resort is cardiac transplantation.

Myocarditis

Aetiopathogenesis

Numerous causes exist for the development of myocarditis. These include RNA and DNA based viruses (coxsackie/ echovirus, poliovirus, respiratory syncytial virus, mumps, adenovirus, Epstein Barr, herpes) bacterial agents such as chlamydia, legionella, mycobacterium, salmonella, streptococcus, fungal and protozoa agents. Additional triggering causes from a non infectious perspective comprise autoimmune disease such as IBD/ rheumatoid arthritis, drugs eg aminophylline, catecholamines, benzodiazepines, diuretics, tetracyclines, penicillin, chemotherapy agents and anti hypertensives

The pathological changes that occur focus on myocyte or matrix based damage. Cytokine release from macrophages follows along with activation of natural killer cells that directly kill cardiac cells infected by infectious agents resulting in further lesion occurrence and impaired function. Overtime leucocytes attempt to clear pathogenic elements. Further cardiac damage however can occur through activation of TGF β and fibrosis formation.

Symptoms

Chest pain
Fever
Sweats
Shortness of breath

Joint discomfort

Palpitations

Syncope

General respiratory or GI symptoms may precede the onset of myocarditis

Signs

Signs are allied to associated heart failure

Differentials

Cardiac tamponade

Cardiogenic shock

Coronary artery disease

HOCM

Cardiomyopathy

Investigations

An ECG is likely to show ischaemic changes with ST segment/ T wave changes and pathological Q waves. There may be elevations in troponin T and I which are more greatly elevated than creatinine kinase MB. There may also be elevations in the ESR, CRP and leucocyte count. Viral antibody titres are also valuable screening tests. An ECHO can help to demonstrate abnormalities such as ventricular dysfunction and thrombi. Cardiac MRI allows for further imaging enhancement demonstrating evidence of oedema and fibrosis. An endomyocardial biopsy (EMB) should be undertaken in patients with heart failure and a normal sized or dilated left ventricle, with less than 2 weeks of symptoms and haemodynamic instability.

Management

The management of myocarditis relies first and foremost on symptom control following the standard treatment pathway of heart failure in the first instance. For viral clearance the utilisation of interferon beta based therapy is essential. Side effects include flu like symptoms and fatigue. Additional treatments include anti inflammatory/ immunosuppressive agents namely immunoglobulins, steroids, azathioprine and cyclosporine.

Rheumatic Fever

Aetiopathogenesis

Group A beta haemolytic streptococcus is the primary agent responsible for rheumatic fever. Molecular mimicry has a strong pathological basis for this condition with a combined humoral and cell mediated response in relation to the bacterium's antigens. This leads to a cross reaction with human cardiac, joint, nervous system and skin tissues. Other agents of concern include Streptococcus pyogenes M type 18.

Symptoms

Sore throat
Joint pain, typically large joint based and symmetrical
Symptoms allied to cardiac dysfunction (carditis — shortness of breath, orthopnoea, chest pain)
Movement dysfunction
Personality changes
Muscle weakness
Speech disorders
Fever

Signs

Swelling, redness and tenderness of the joints
Cardiac signs, namely murmurs (such as mitral and aortic regurgitation), friction rubs, evidence of heart failure
Subcutaneous nodules
Erythema marginatum

Differentials

Septic arthritis

Connective tissue disease

Lyme disease

Infective endocarditis

Sickle cell anaemia

Lymphoma

Leukaemia

Major criteria

- Carditis
- Polyarthritis
- Subcutaneous nodules
- Erythema marginatum
- Chorea

Minor criteria

- Prolonged PR interval on electrocardiogram
- Arthralgia
- Fever
- Acute phase reactants: raised erythrocyte sedimentation rate or raised C reactive protein levels
- Plus supporting evidence of a preceding streptococcal infection for both major and minor criteria

Investigations

The modified Jones criteria above aids in the diagnosis of rheumatic fever, with a focus on two major manifestations or one major and two minor, alongside an increase in anti streptolysin O. Imaging relies on the use of an ECHO which helps to demonstrate valvular abnormalities, impaired left ventricular function or an end systolic diameter of 40 mm or greater. Additional blood investigations include inflammatory markers (CRP and ESR) as well as blood cultures. A throat culture for group A streptococcus is advised.

Management

Evidence for the treatment of rheumatic fever is not overwhelming. Therapies from a medical perspective include anti inflammatory agents, steroids and antibiotics namely penicillin. Surgical repair and replacement of valvular dysfunction is also advised.

Peripheral Arterial Disease

Aetiopathogenesis

Risk factors for the development of peripheral arterial disease comprise diabetes, smoking, hypertension and hypercholesterolaemia. An inflammatory process is the primary trigger disease wise with selectin adhesion molecules aiding in the deposition of leucocytes on the endothelium. Two groups of selectin adhesion molecules include P selectin and vascular cell adhesion protein 1. As leucocytes accumulate they gather lipids and appear foam like in nature. Overtime transformation to a more advanced plaque occurs with deposition of muscle cells, collagen and calcium leading to a more fibrous nature. Plaque stability can be impaired secondary to inflammation and metalloproteinases which digest collagen. Elastin break down is also a common occurrence courtesy of cathepsin S and K. Smooth muscle breakdown can also take place via apoptosis. Platelets and fibrinogen later form a platelet plug leading to vessel obstruction immediately or further downstream.

Symptoms

Pain precipitated by walking and relieved by rest
Impotence in males

Signs

Absent pulses
Paralysis
Pain

Skin pallor/ atrophy/ dry scaly appearance/ hair loss/ ulceration
Paraesthesia
Livedo reticularis

Differentials
Thrombophlebitis
Deep Vein Thrombosis

Investigations
One of the primary investigations of choice is the ankle brachial pressure index whilst the patient is supine. Systolic blood pressure measurement in both arms as well as the posterior tibial/ dorsalis pedis/ peroneal pulse is necessary. The index in each leg is determined by dividing the highest ankle pressure by the highest arm pressure.

Imaging relies on the use of duplex ultrasound in addition to CT/ MRI angiography.

Management
Management of intermittent claudication relies on regular exercise based intervention and risk factor modification. Further treatment relies on the use of angioplasty and primary stent therapies for patients with complete aorto iliac occlusion. If angioplasty fails then consideration for bypass surgery is the next stage. If patients resist either angioplasty or bypass based intervention evidence suggests the use of the vasodilator naftidrofuryl oxalate.

Critical limb ischaemia management focuses on angioplasty or bypass surgery with stent placement for patients with critical limb ischaemia secondary to aorto iliac occlusion. Pain requires the utilisation of opioids and paracetamol.

Atrial Fibrillation

Aetiopathogenesis

Various factors are responsible for the occurrence of atrial fibrillation (AF). These include valvular heart disease, coronary artery disease, diabetes, obesity, hypertension, endocrine dysfunction, congestive cardiac failure, alcohol, illicit drug use, respiratory disorders, neurological events such as a stroke and infection. The exact focus for AF is not known. It is assumed to be pulmonary vein related. It is also assumed that maintenance of atrial fibrillation relies on atrial restructuring and electrical remodelling.

Symptoms

Chest pain
Palpitations
Shortness of breath
Fatigue
Weakness
Syncope

Signs

Irregularly irregular pulse — tachy or bradycardia may be present
Evidence of underlying disease (neurological/ endocrine for example)

Differentials

Atrial flutter
Supraventricular tachycardia
Wolff-Parkinson-White syndrome

Investigations

An ECG is of course required. For patients with suspected paroxysmal AF then a 24 hour ECG monitor is preferred. A transthoracic ECHO is also of value with progression to a trans oesophageal ECHO if a TTE has been problematic. The CHA_2DS_2-VASc score is advised in order to assess the risk of stroke in patients with AF.

Age	<65 0	65-74 +1	≥75 +2
Sex	Female +1		Male 0
Congestive heart failure history	No 0		Yes +1
Hypertension history	No 0		Yes +1
Stroke/TIA/Thromboembolism history	No 0		Yes +2
Vascular disease history	No 0		Yes +1
Diabetes history	No 0		Yes +1

Management

Anticoagulation is advised for patients with a CHA_2DS_2-VASc of 1 if male or for all individuals if greater than 2. Suitable agents of choice include apixaban, dabigatran, rivaroxaban or a vitamin K antagonist. Note that bleeding is an obvious risk and must be taken into account.

Rate control is the typical treatment of choice for patients. This includes a β blocker (bar sotalol) or a calcium channel blocker. Combination therapies can also be attempted comprising a β blocker, diltiazem or digoxin. Rhythm control is employed where rate control has failed to resolve the issue. Electrical cardioversion is advised for those patients where AF has remained for greater than 48 hours. Amiodarone should be commenced prior to and after electrical cardioversion. Long term rhythm control agents include β blockers and dronedarone.

Patients with infrequent symptoms and paroxysms should be treated via the highly regarded 'pill in the pocket' regimen. If drug intervention has not been successful or is contraindicated then left atrial catheter ablation is the next stage.

Acute Management

Emergency electrical cardioversion is advised in those who are presenting with haemodynamic instability. Within a 48 hour presentation without haemodynamic concerns, rate or rhythm control is advised. If the presentation is typically greater than 48 hours then rate control is preferred.

Pharmacological cardioversion focuses on the use of flecanide for those patients without structural or ischaemic heart pathology. Amiodarone is preferred in those with evidence of structural heart damage. If the period of AF is assumed longer than 48 hours, cardioversion should be halted until anticoagulation has occurred for three weeks.

Preferred anti coagulation is heparin initially. Oral anti coagulation is then commenced in those with recent onset AF if stable sinus rhythm has not been restored and risk of recurrence is high.

Arrhythmias

For the purpose of real life clinical practice this section focuses on the management strategies for arrhythmias in reference to Advanced Life Support UK. A more detailed overview would be needed if pursing higher cardiology training.

Tachycardia

The management approach for patients with tachycardia is indicated below. For patients requiring synchronised cardioversion, sedation / general anaesthesia is needed.

- For a broad-complex tachycardia or atrial fibrillation, start with 120–150 J and increase in increments
- For atrial flutter and regular narrow-complex tachycardia start with 70–120 J

The management of AF has been described in detail previously.

Bradycardia

The management of bradycardia is indicated below.

In a clinical setting awareness of the possible causes of arrhythmias are relevant. Examples include:

Bradycardia — drugs such as calcium channel blockers, beta blockers, digoxin, amiodarone, sick sinus syndrome, hypothermia, hypoglycaemia

Tachycardia — ischaemic heart disease, congenital heart disease, cardiomyopathies, channelopathies, electrolyte dysfunction (eg hypokalaemia/hypocalcaemia), drugs such as cocaine and rheumatological conditions (RA/SLE)

Assess using the ABCDE approach
- Monitor SpO$_2$ and give oxygen if hypoxic
- Monitor ECG and BP, and record 12-lead ECG
- Obtain IV access
- Identify and treat reversible causes (e.g. electrolyte abnormalities)

Adverse features?
- Shock
- Syncope
- Myocardial ischaemia
- Heart failure

Is QRS narrow (< 0.12 s)?

Yes - Unstable

Synchronised DC Shock*
Up to 3 attempts

Seek expert help

- Amiodarone 300 mg IV over 10-20 min
- Repeat shock
- Then give amiodarone 900 mg over 24 h

No - Stable

Broad

Broad QRS
Is QRS regular?

Regular

- If VT (or uncertain rhythm):
  Amiodarone 300 mg IV over 20-60 min then 900 mg over 24 h
- If known to be SVT with bundle branch block:
  Treat as for regular narrow-complex tachycardia

Irregular

Seek expert help

Possibilities include:
- AF with bundle branch block treat as for narrow complex
- Pre-excited AF consider amiodarone

Narrow

Narrow QRS
Is rhythm regular?

Regular

- Vagal manoeuvres
- Adenosine 6 mg rapid IV bolus
  If no effect give 12 mg
  If no effect give further 12 mg
  Monitor/record ECG continuously

Sinus rhythm achieved?

Yes

Probable re-entry paroxysmal SVT:
- Record 12-lead ECG in sinus rhythm
- If SVT recurs treat again and consider anti-arrhythmic prophylaxis

No

Seek expert help

Irregular

Probable AF:
- Control rate with beta-blocker or diltiazem
- If in heart failure consider digoxin or amiodarone
- Assess thromboembolic risk and consider anticoagulation

Seek expert help

Possible atrial flutter:
- Control rate (e.g. with beta-blocker)

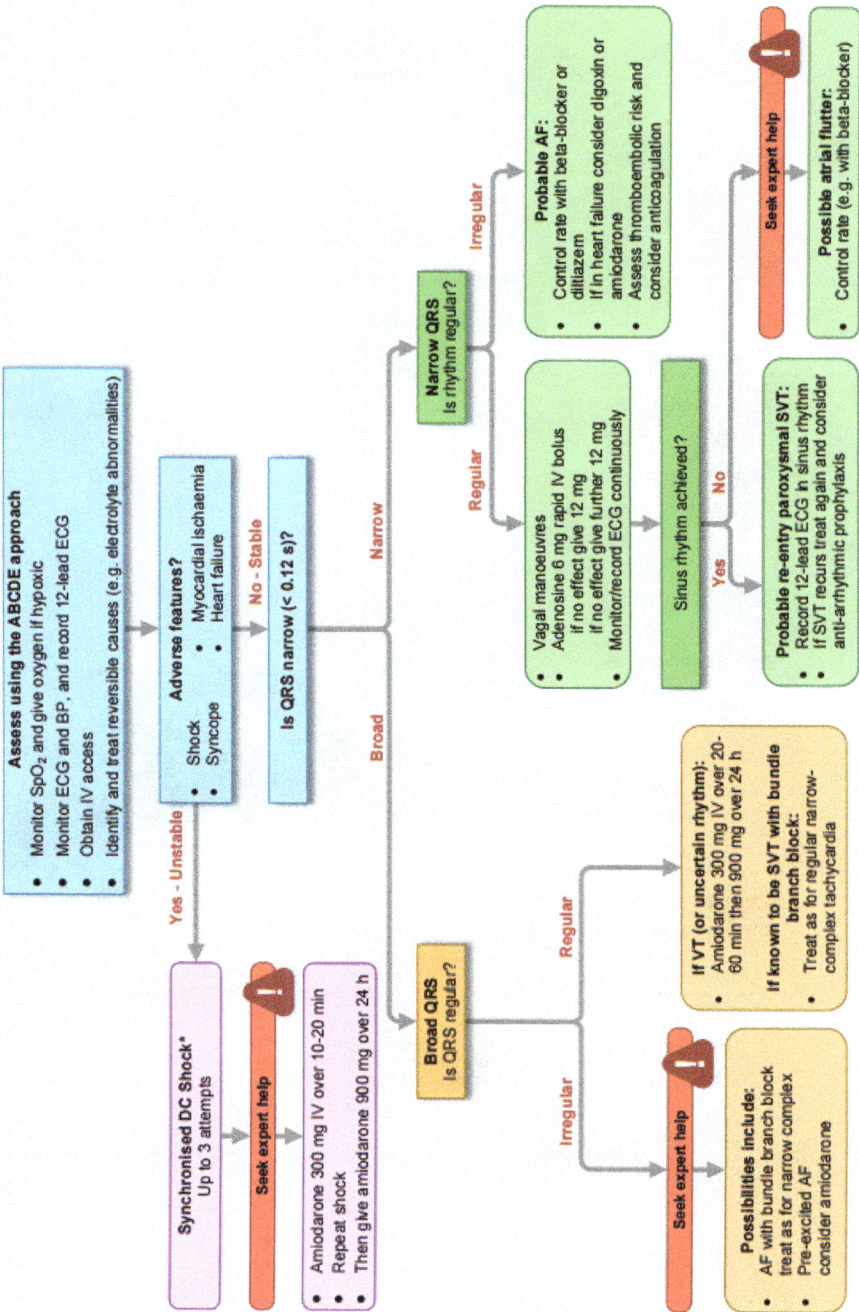

*Conscious patients require sedation or general anaesthesia for cardioversion

Assess using the ABCDE approach
- Monitor SpO$_2$ and give oxygen if hypoxic
- Monitor ECG and BP, and record 12-lead ECG
- Obtain IV access
- Identify and treat reversible causes (e.g. electrolyte abnormalities)

Adverse features?
- Shock
- Syncope
- Myocardial ischaemia
- Heart failure

Yes ← → No

Atropine 500 mcg IV

Satisfactory response?

No ← → Yes

Consider interim measures:
- Atropine 500 mcg IV repeat to maximum of 3 mg
  OR
- Transcutaneous pacing
  OR
- Isoprenaline 5 mcg min^{-1} IV
- Adrenaline 2-10 mcg min^{-1} IV
- Alternative drugs*

← Yes

Risk of asystole?
- Recent asystole
- Mobitz II AV block
- Complete heart block with broad QRS
- Ventricular pause > 3 s

No

Seek expert help
Arrange transvenous pacing

Continue observation

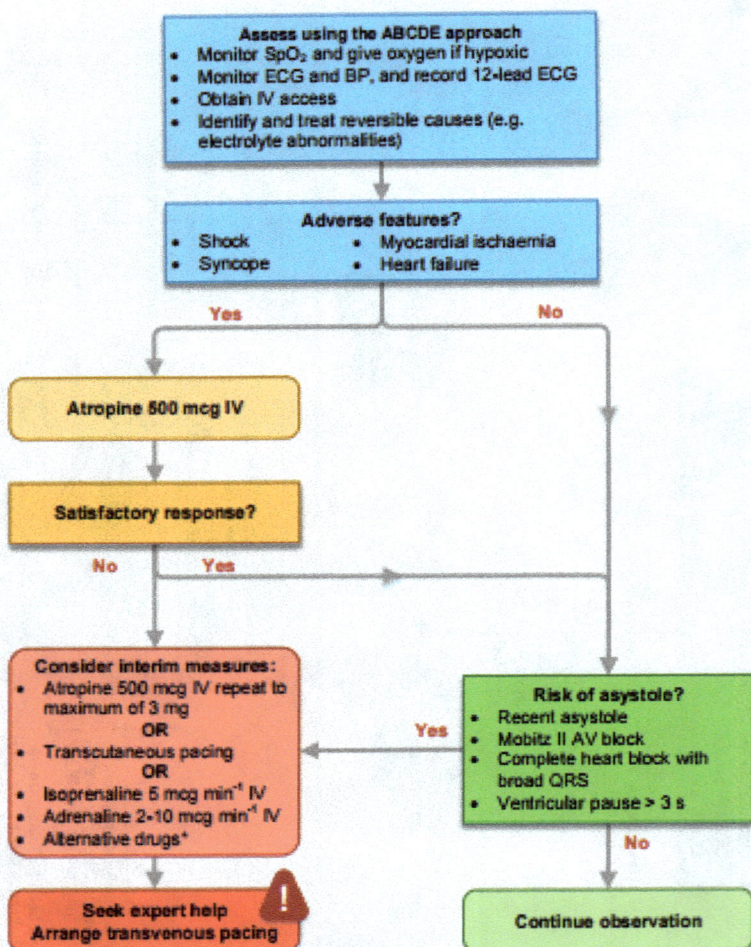

* Alternatives include:
- Aminophylline
- Dopamine
- Glucagon (if bradycardia is caused by beta-blocker or calcium channel blocker)
- Glycopyrrolate (may be used instead of atropine)

A Note on Congenital Heart Disease

A detailed understanding of congenital heart disease (CHD) is required during higher specialist training. For early working life as a doctor a broad based overview is sufficient.

Atrial septal defect (ASD) — right sided heart dilatation occurs in this instance secondary to a hole in the atrial septum and blood shunting from the left to the right atrium. Various types exist: secundum (most common, located in the middle of the wall between the atria), primum (lowest portion of the atrial septum), sinus venosus (upper part of the atrial septum) and coronary sinus (a part of the wall between the coronary sinus and left atrium is missing). Examination findings highlight a fixed and widely split S2 along with an ejection systolic murmur and ejection click. Treatment relies on percutaneous or surgical closure. And post closure one must be aware of an increased risk of AF, stroke and heart failure.

Ventricular septal defect (VSD) — associated with blood shunting from the left to the right ventricle. Infective endocarditis is a common drawback in such instances. In addition there is a risk of Eisenmenger's syndrome which is linked to elevated pulmonary vascular resistance, shunt reversal and desaturation. Examination findings typically highlight a pansystolic murmur at the left sternal edge.

Patent ductus arteriosus — a connection between the pulmonary artery and aorta which is present in the foetal circulation and can lead to left ventricular dilatation. A continuous murmur on auscultation is evident with closure typically achieved percutaneously.

Coarctation of the aorta — here narrowing of the aorta distal to the origin of the left subclavian artery is noted. Notable hypertension exists with absent femoral pulses. Stenting is often the treatment of choice.

Tetralogy of Fallot — right ventricular (RV) outflow tract obstruction (RVOTO) (infundibular stenosis), ventricular septal defect (VSD), aorta dextroposition, and right ventricular hypertrophy. Management relies on patch closure of the VSD, resection of the infundibular stenosis and patch augmentation of the RVOTO. Pulmonary valve implantation is often required due to resulting pulmonary regurgitation.

Transposition of the great arteries — here the aorta arises from the right ventricle and the pulmonary artery from the left. The intervention of choice is the arterial switch where the great vessels are transposed and the native pulmonary valve becomes the valve for systemic outflow and the aortic valve becomes the valve for outflow to the pulmonary artery.

It is important to note that post repair of CHD there is a risk of subsequent infective endocarditis and hence antibiotic prophylaxis is often recommended yet the debate continues as to its widespread adoption.

Various risk factors exist for the development of CHD and include maternal diabetes, rubella, drugs such as lithium, alcohol and isotretinoin as well as genetic factors. Down's syndrome is a common genetic syndrome associated with CHD.

The symptoms of CHD that are known to be of concern include:

- Progressive or paroxysmal breathlessness—consider new onset of arrhythmia
- Palpitations—consider new arrhythmia or deteriorating valve or ventricular function
- Fevers, malaise, weight loss—consider infective endocarditis until proved otherwise
- Rapidly increasing weight or peripheral oedema—consider arrhythmias or heart failure

For women seeking contraceptive advice, current recommendations focus on progesterone only contraceptives due to the increased risk of thromboembolism in CHD. Hence oestrogen contraceptives are best avoided.

Investigations

Investigations of choice include a TTE or TOE. Further imaging relies on CT or MRI as well as cardiac catheterisation. Imaging in general allows for the assessment of ventricular function, haemodynamics and valvular function.

Examination Skills

Introduction

Effective examination skills are key to determining a diagnosis alongside an accurate history. During medical school and early junior doctor years the assessment of examination skills during an OSCE or postgraduate examination setting is something feared by most, if not all. Regardless of this fact it is important to note that there are only a finite number of stations that can appear. What you must remember is that the mark schemes at either an undergraduate/ postgraduate level are universal. Examiners are expecting you to demonstrate an appropriate rapport with the patient in the first instance being mindful of any concerns they may have during the examination. In addition, candidates should be able to perform a thorough and systematic systems examination and be prepared to detect physical signs, construct differentials and detail potential investigation and management strategies. Each station is schema dependent, so be weary of preferred presentation style. For example, an examiner may simply ask you to palpate the abdomen. In addition some may prefer you not to talk through your examination as you perform it. You can imagine how laborious it becomes for them when the candidate begins as follows: 'I am standing at the end of the bed and observing for any scars or masses... I am now looking at the hands for clubbing etc etc...' It may seem that they are rushing you through but that is so they can reach all station aspects and ensure you can gain as many points as possible.

The following cases are all likely at an undergraduate and postgraduate level, some harder than others. However if faced with difficulty keep things simple and DO NOT invent signs. Examiners are quick to spot the actor type candidate and this will not bode well in terms of professionalism/ probity. Be observant of the fact that you are only likely to face a two to three minute interplay with the examiner post examination so follow the pattern of signs, differentials, investigations and management and make sure to keep it sharp and most of all simple. Examiners get frustrated with long drawn out negatives and several random causes which are not applicable to pathology in the UK. In other words an opening discussion could be something along the following lines... ' On examination the patient appears comfortable/distressed. There is evidence of x, y and z. The most likely diagnosis is... secondary to x, y and z.'

Or

'I am unsure of the diagnosis but would like to offer the following differentials. In order to obtain a diagnosis I would undertake the following tests.'

Start with blood investigations before imaging. And if you are 100% convinced of the diagnosis then offer a management plan. OK, on to the cases!

Valvular Heart Disease

The most common OSCE scenario in cardiology is centred on valvular heart disease. Examiners will ask for underlying causes, investigations and management details accordingly. There may also be patients with mixed valve disease!

Aetiology

Causes of valvular heart disease are numerous and include:

Aortic regurgitation	— connective tissue disease eg RA, infective endocarditis, hypertension, bicuspid aortic valve
Aortic stenosis	— congenital, Rheumatic fever, bicuspid aortic valve, calcification, infective endocarditis, hyperuricaemia, Paget's disease
Mitral regurgitation	— Rheumatic fever, connective tissue dysfunction, ruptured chordae tendineae, annular dilatation, infective endocarditis
Mitral stenosis	— congenital, connective tissue dysfunction eg SLE
Tricuspid regurgitation	— Rheumatic fever, infective endocarditis, connective tissue disease, Ebstein's anomaly (valve leaflet displacement)
Tricuspid stenosis	— Rheumatic fever, carcinoid syndrome, infective endocarditis, connective tissue disease

Symptoms

In general the symptoms of patients with valvular heart disease comprise:

Chest pain
Palpitations
Shortness of breath

Fatigue
Breathlessness when lying flat
Syncope

Signs

AR

Early diastolic murmur left sternal border best heard with the patient sitting forward in expiration, wide pulse pressures, collapsing 'water hammer' pulse, visible pulsations in the fingernails, head bobbing with each heartbeat, uvula pulsations, retinal arteriole pulsations, 'pistol shot' or booming sounds noted over the femoral artery along with apex beat displacement.

AS

Slow rising pulse, narrow pulse pressure, soft S2 with splitting of S2, S4, pulsus alternans, ejection systolic murmur radiating to the carotids.

MR

Diminished first heart sound, S3, blowing murmur at the apex radiating to the axilla, pansystolic in nature.

MS

Mitral facies, atrial fibrillation, loud first heart sound, tapping apex, opening snap, diastolic rumbling murmur best heard in the left lateral position in expiration.

TR

Elevated JVP, S3, pan systolic murmur high pitched and augmented during inspiration.

TS

Diastolic murmur left sternal border which enhances during inspiration, splitting of the first heart sound.

It is important to note that when presenting any patient with valvular heart disease, mentioning evidence of pulmonary hypertension or heart failure is essential. And always remember to assess the pulse!

Investigations

Investigations of choice include a TTE and a TOE when the former is suboptimal in nature. Additional investigations of value include stress testing, exercise ECG/ ECHO and cardiac magnetic resonance/ CT. It is important to note that ECHO findings typically help in aiding management.

Management

In reference to the current guidelines the following management is indicated:

Surgery is indicated in symptomatic patients.

Surgery is indicated in asymptomatic patients with a resting left ventricular ejection fraction ≤50%.

Surgery is indicated in patients undergoing CABG or surgery of the ascending aorta.

Surgery should be considered in asymptomatic patients with a resting EF >50% with severe LV dilatation: Left Ventricular End Diastolic Diameter >70 mm, or LV end-systolic diameter >50 mm

Aortic Root Disease

Surgery is indicated in patients who have aortic root disease with maximal ascending aortic diameter ≥50 mm for patients with Marfan syndrome.

Surgery should be considered in patients who have aortic root disease with a maximal ascending aortic diameter: ≥45 mm for patients with Marfan syndrome with risk factors, ≥50 mm for patients with bicuspid valve with risk factors or ≥55 mm for other patients.

Aortic stenosis — aortic valve replacement is indicated in patients with severe AS and any symptoms related to AS.

AVR is indicated in patients with severe AS undergoing CABG, surgery of the ascending aorta or of another valve.

AVR is indicated in asymptomatic patients with severe AS and systolic LV dysfunction (LVEF <50%) not due to another cause.

AVR is indicated in asymptomatic patients with severe AS and abnormal exercise test showing symptoms on exercise clearly related to AS.

AVR should be considered in high risk patients with severe symptomatic AS who are suitable for transcatheter aortic valve implantation, but in whom surgery is favoured by a 'heart team' based on the individual risk profile.

AVR should be considered in asymptomatic patients with severe AS and an abnormal exercise test showing a fall in blood pressure below baseline.

AVR should be considered in patients with moderate AS undergoing CABG, surgery of the ascending aorta or of another valve.

AVR should be considered in symptomatic patients with low flow, low gradient (<40 mmHg) AS with normal EF only after careful confirmation of severe AS.

AVR should be considered in symptomatic patients with severe AS, low flow, low gradient with reduced EF, and evidence of flow reserve.

AVR should be considered in asymptomatic patients, with normal EF and none of the above mentioned exercise test abnormalities, if the surgical risk is low, and one or more of the following findings is present: Very severe AS defined by a peak transvalvular velocity >5.5 m/s or, severe valve calcification and a rate of peak transvalvular velocity progression ≥0.3 m/s per year.

AVR may be considered in symptomatic patients with severe AS low flow, low gradient, and LV dysfunction without flow reserve.

AVR may be considered in asymptomatic patients with severe AS, normal EF and none of the above mentioned exercise test abnormalities, if surgical risk is low, and one or more of the following findings is present: Markedly elevated natriuretic peptide levels confirmed by repeated measurements and without other explanations, increase of mean pressure gradient with exercise by >20 mmHg, excessive LV hypertrophy in the absence of hypertension.

Mitral Regurgitation

Mitral valve repair should be the preferred technique when it is expected to be durable.

Surgery is indicated in symptomatic patients with LVEF>30% and LVESD < 55mm.

Surgery is indicated in asymptomatic patients with LV dysfunction (LVESD ≥45 mm and/or LVEF ≤60%).

Surgery should be considered in asymptomatic patients with preserved LV function and new onset of atrial fibrillation or pulmonary hypertension (systolic pulmonary pressure at rest >50 mmHg).

Surgery should be considered in asymptomatic patients with preserved LV function, high likelihood of durable repair, low surgical risk and flail leaflet and LVESD ≥40 mm.

Surgery should be considered in patients with severe LV dysfunction (LVEF <30 % and/ or LVESD>55mm) refractory to medical therapy with high/low likelihood of durable repair and low comorbidity.

Surgery may be considered in asymptomatic patients with preserved LV function, high likelihood of durable repair, low surgical risk and: left atrial dilatation (volume index ≥60 ml/m^2 BSA) and sinus rhythm, or pulmonary hypertension (see below for an overview of pulmonary hypertension) on exercise (systolic pulmonary artery pressure ≥60 mmHg at exercise).

Mitral Stenosis

Percutaneous mitral commissurotomy is indicated in symptomatic patients with favourable characteristics.

PMC is indicated in symptomatic patients with a contraindication or high risk for surgery.

PMC should be considered as initial treatment in symptomatic patients with unfavourable anatomy but without unfavourable clinical characteristics.

PMC should be considered in asymptomatic patients without unfavourable characteristics and a high thromboembolic risk (previous history of embolism, dense spontaneous contrast in the left atrium, recent or paroxysmal atrial fibrillation) and/or high risk of haemodynamic decompensation (systolic pulmonary pressure >50 mmHg at rest, need for major non-cardiac surgery, desire for pregnancy).

Tricuspid Valve Disease

Surgery is indicated in symptomatic patients with severe TS. Surgery is indicated in patients with severe TS undergoing left-sided valve intervention. Surgery is indicated in patients with severe primary or secondary TR undergoing left-sided valve surgery. Surgery is indicated in symptomatic patients with severe isolated primary TR without severe right ventricular dysfunction. Surgery should be considered in patients with moderate primary TR undergoing left-sided valve surgery. Surgery should be considered in patients with mild or moderate secondary TR with a dilated annulus (≥40 mm or >21 mm/m²) undergoing left-sided valve surgery. Surgery should be considered in asymptomatic or mildly symptomatic patients with severe isolated primary TR and progressive right ventricular dilatation or deterioration of right ventricular function. After left-sided valve surgery, surgery should be considered in patients with severe TR who are symptomatic or have progressive right ventricular dilatation/dysfunction, in the absence of left-sided valve dysfunction, severe right or left ventricular dysfunction, and severe pulmonary vascular disease.

It is important to note that in view of resulting heart failure, medical therapies as discussed earlier should be considered.

In general, the choice of valve replacement, be it mechanical or bio prosthetic, relies on the need for anticoagulation. If anticoagulation will be problematic, due to compliance or bleeding risk, a bioprosthesis is more suitable. A target INR of 3-4 is advised when anticoagulation is utilised.

In the OSCE, patients with valvular replacement may be potential cases. The obvious give away is the presence of a scar and audible click. The examination aspect is relatively quick in this regard and the discussion will focus more on indications for valve replacement, choice of valve as highlighted above and potential complications. These include endocarditis, thromboembolism, valvular failure and bleeding.

An Overview of Pulmonary Hypertension

PH is defined as an increase in mean pulmonary arterial pressure (PAPm) ≥25 mmHg at rest as assessed by right heart catheterization (RHC). Numerous causes exist including genetic mutations, drugs such as anorectics, left sided heart disease, lung disease, connective tissue dysfunction, HIV, haematological and metabolic disorders. Patients typically present with shortness of breath, fatigue, angina and syncope. On examination notable signs include a left parasternal lift, accentuation of the pulmonary aspect of the second heart sound, a pan systolic murmur of tricuspid regurgitation and a diastolic murmur of pulmonary regurgitation (note that this is secondary to pulmonary hypertension and primary causes can include infective endocarditis, rheumatic fever and carcinoid syndrome). An elevated JVP, hepatomegaly, ascites and peripheral oedema are notable. Investigations of choice include an ECG which can indicate right ventricular hypertrophy and right bundle branch block. Further investigations of choice include a chest X ray, pulmonary function tests indicative of lung volume reduction, echocardiography to typically assess tricuspid regurgitation velocity and elevated right sided heart pressures, ventilation perfusion/CT pulmonary angiogram imaging to determine the existence of thromboembolic pulmonary disease as well as cardiac magnetic resonance imaging, right heart catheterisation and vasoreactivity testing.

Management relies on enhanced physical activity, oxygen use for those patients with a pO_2 < 8 kPa, diuretics, calcium channel blockers, endothelin receptor antagonists such as bosentan/ ambrisentan, phosphodiesterase type 5 inhibitors such as sildenafil and prostacyclin analogues such as epoprostenol. Failure of maximal medical therapy relies on lung transplantation or balloon atrial septostomy.

ECGs

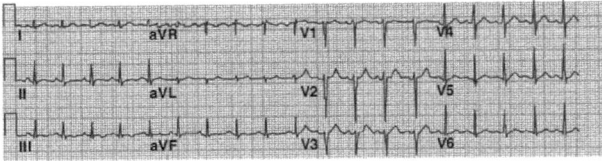

Sinus tachycardia

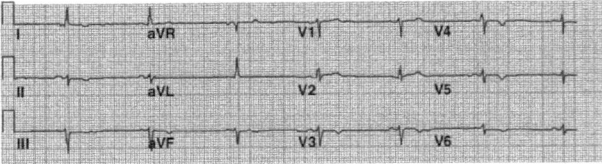

Sinus bradycardia

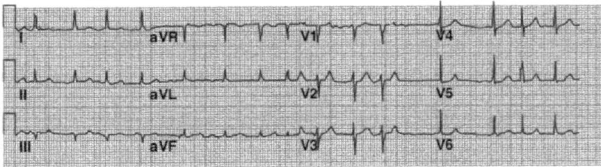

Atrial fibrillation

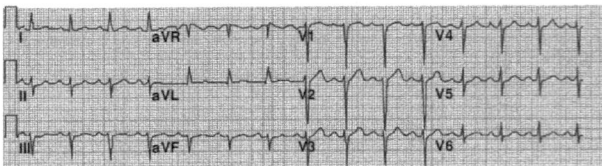

First degree Heart Block

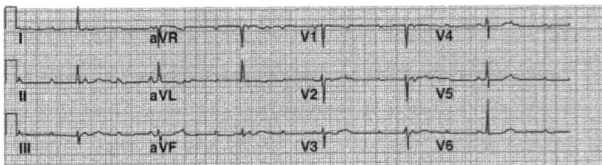

Complete Heart Block

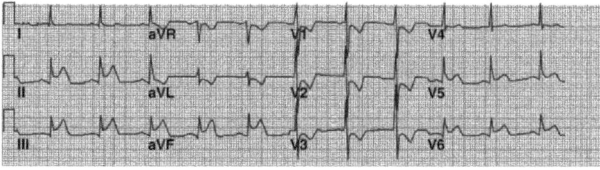

Inferior Posterior MI

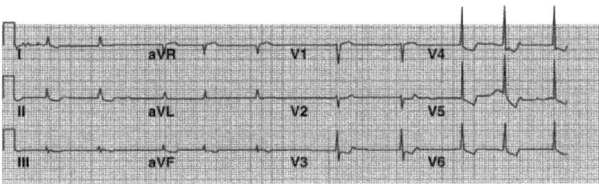

Digoxin toxicity

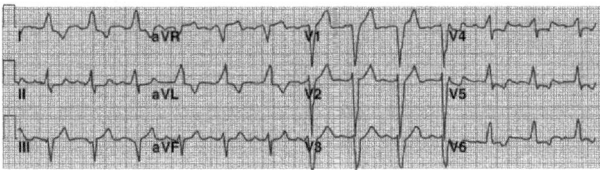

Left Bundle Branch Block

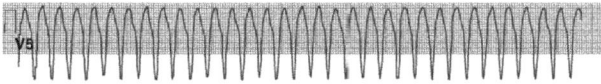

Ventricular tachycardia

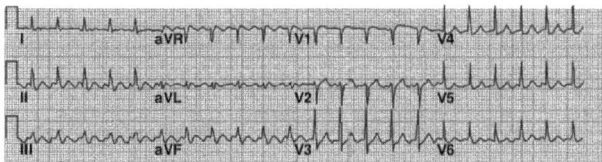

Atrial flutter

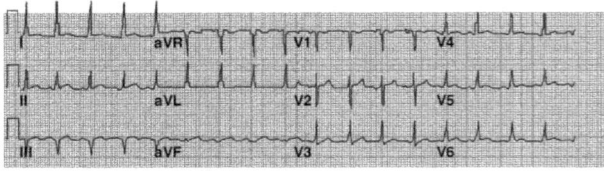

Wolff Parkinson White syndrome

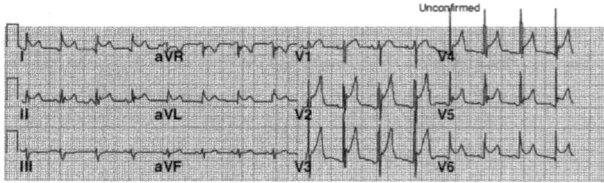

Pericarditis

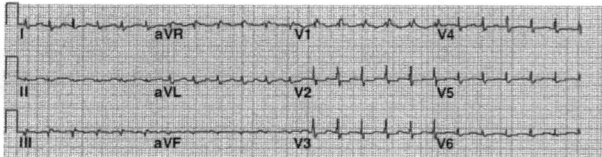

Low voltage complexes

References

Acute Coronary Syndrome. SIGN. Available from www.sign.ac.uk/assets/sign148.pdf

Acute Heart Failure Diagnosis and Management. NICE Guidelines. Available from https://www.nice.org.uk/guidance/cg187/resources/acute-heart-failure-diagnosis-and-management-35109817738693

Chronic Heart Failure in Adults: Management. NICE Guidelines. Available from https://www.nice.org.uk/guidance/cg108/resources/chronic-heart-failure-in-adults-management-35109335688901

Classes of Heart Failure. Available from http://www.heart.org/HEARTORG/Conditions/HeartFailure/AboutHeartFailure/Classes-of-Heart-Failure_UCM_306328_Article.jsp#.WocFCVoiIdV

Dwornik M. Circulatory Support in Cardiogenic Shock: A Focused Update for a General Cardiologist. Available from https://www.bcs.com/pages/news_full.asp?NewsID=19792461

Elliot CA, Kiely DG. Pulmonary hypertension. *Br J Anaes* 2006;6(1):17–22, https://doi.org/10.1093/bjaceaccp/mki061

Gould FK, Denning DW, Elliott TS *et al.* Guidelines for the diagnosis and antibiotic treatment of endocarditis in adults: a report of the Working Party of the British Society for Antimicrobial Chemotherapy. *J Antimicrob Chemother.* 2012;67(2):269–289, doi: 10.1093/jac/dkr450 (Epub 2011 Nov 14).

Grace 2.0 Risk Calculator. Available from http://gracescore.org/WebSite/Default.aspx

Guidelines on the Diagnosis and Management of Pericardial Diseases. Executive Summary. Available from http://www.escardio.org/static_file/Escardio/Guidelines/publications/ PERICAguidelines-pericardial-ES.pdf

Hypertension in Adults: Diagnosis and Management. NICE Guidelines. Available from https://www.nice.org.uk/guidance/cg127/chapter/1-Guidance#measuring blood-pressure

Implantable Cardioverter Defibrillators and Cardiac Resynchronisation Therapy for Arrhythmias and Heart Failure. NICE Guidelines. Available from https://www.nice.org.uk/guidance/ta314/chapter/1-Guidance

Kushwaha SS, Falon JT, Fuster V. Restrictive cardiomyopathy. *N Engl J Med* 1997;336:267–276, doi: 10.1056/NEJM199701233360407.

Luk A, Ahn E, Soor GS *et al.* Dilated cardiomyopathy: a review. *J Clin Pathol.* 2009;62(3):219–225, doi: 10.1136/jcp.2008.060731 (Epub 2008 Nov 18).

Maron B *et al.* Hypertrophic cardiomyopathy. *Lancet* 2013;381(9862):242–255.

Moreillon P. Infective endocarditis. *Lancet* 2004;363(9403):139–149.

Ouriel K. Peripheral arterial disease. *Lancet* 2001;358(9289):1257–1264.

Pandya B, Cullen S, Walker F. Congenital heart disease in adults. *Br Med J* 2016;354:i3905.

Peripheral Arterial Disease: Diagnosis and Management. NICE Guidelines. Available from https://www.nice.org.uk/guidance/CG147/chapter/1-Guidance# diagnosis

Schultheiss H-P, Kühl U, Cooper LT. The management of myocarditis. *Eur Heart J* 2011;32(21):2616–2625, https://doi.org/10.1093/eurheartj/ehr165

Shah A *et al.* In search of new therapeutic targets and strategies for heart failure: recent advances in basic science. *Lancet* 2011;378(9792):704–712.

Stable Angina: Management. NICE Guidelines. Available from https://www.nice.org.uk/guidance/cg126/resources/stable-angina-management- 35109453262021

Valvular Heart Disease (Management of). ESC Clinical Practice Guidelines. Available from https://www.escardio.org/Guidelines/Clinical-Practice-Guidelines/Valvular-Heart-Disease-Management-of

Webb RH, Grant C, Harnden A. Acute rheumatic fever. *Br Med J* 2015;351:h3443.

Disclaimer

This text was produced in reference to current guidelines. At the time of publication there may have been further updates to the evidence and the reader is advised to be aware of this fact. Furthermore any drugs listed may or may not have drug dosages listed to minimise potential errors. Readers are advised to refer to the latest pharmaceutical formularies for clarification.

Notes

Part III
Respiratory Medicine

Chronic Obstructive Pulmonary Disease (COPD)

Aetiopathogenesis

Smoking has been deemed the primary cause of COPD along with chronic exposure to pollutants. Genetic associations with alpha 1 anti-trypsin (A1AT) deficiency is a notable cause. A1AT is a protease inhibitor neutralising neutrophil elastase and hence its loss leads to significant parenchymal damage. The most common deficiency state is the PiZZ genotype.

COPD demonstrates evidence of airway remodelling which is non reversible in nature with alveolar damage leading to loss of elastic recoil and emphysema based changes. Airway thickening is seen along with smooth muscle and mucus gland hyperplasia with an increased production of inflammatory cells. Toll like receptor activation has been demonstrated particularly 2 and 4 with cytokine release namely Tumour necrosis factor alpha and interleukin 1 and 8. T helper cell activation has been described leading to further proinflammatory developments as well as CD8 T cell involvement. Oxidative stress occurs with cellular apoptosis and fibrosis secondary to Transforming growth factor β. Matrix metalloproteinase formation results in notable lung structural damage. And there is significant macrophage dysfunction impairing apoptotic cell removal. Ciliary damage leads to mucus build up and the excess sputum formation seen in chronic bronchitis.

Symptoms

Cough productive in nature

Shortness of breath

Diminished exercise tolerance

Signs

Wheeze

Diminished breath sounds

Hyperinflated chest

Hyper resonance on chest percussion

Prolongation of expiration

Accessory muscle usage

Evidence of right heart failure (namely cor pulmonale)

Differentials

Bronchitis

Emphysema

Pulmonary embolism

Alpha 1 anti trypsin deficiency

Investigations

Bloods in the first instance are critical particularly an arterial blood gas in view of the risk of type II respiratory failure. A full blood count will help to demonstrate evidence of infection as well as secondary polycythaemia. There may be evidence of a lowered serum potassium in view of bronchodilator use. Patients should undergo sputum screening for microscopy, culture and sensitivity as well as alpha 1 anti trypsin measurement. A chest X ray helps to demonstrate lung hyperinflation as well as the possible presence of bullae. More advanced imaging involves a high resolution CT to screen particularly for bullous based lesions. An ECG should be requested which may help to demonstrate right ventricular hypertrophy. Lung function tests should be performed to confirm an obstructive picture, namely an FEV_1: FVC ratio of less than 70%. Airflow obstruction severity can be determined following bronchodilator intervention.

- FEV_1 > 80% predicted — mild
- 50–79% — moderate
- 30–49% — severe
- < 30% — very severe

Management

Smoking cessation is advised where applicable. Options to assist in such situations comprise nicotine replacement therapy or varenicline. Inhaler based therapy is vital and comprises short acting β2 agonists as well as short acting muscarinic antagonists. Long acting β2 agonists/ long acting muscarinic antagonists are advisable in those who still remain breathless and suffer exacerbations in addition to inhaled steroids. If breathing remains problematic despite such interventions then nebulised therapy is advised. Oral theophylline can be employed in patients who have failed long acting bronchodilators and are unable to utilise inhaled therapies overall. Mucolytics should be given to patients with productive sputum. For patients with a pO_2 less than 7.3 kPa or one less than 8 kPa with polycythaemia, nocturnal hypoxia, peripheral oedema or pulmonary hypertension, long term oxygen therapy is recommended for a minimum of 15 hours per day. Those keen to continue with oxygen therapy outside their home should be prescribed ambulatory oxygen accordingly. Non invasive ventilation should be considered in those patients with hypercapnic respiratory failure. Pulmonary rehabilitation should be offered to COPD patients who score 3 or higher on the MRC dyspnoea scale (3 — stops for breath when walking at own pace, 4 — stops for breath after walking 100 m, 5 — too breathless to leave their home).

Surgical intervention in COPD patients is advised for those with a single bulla on CT and an FEV_1 < 50% predicted. Lung volume reduction surgery is appropriate for those with an FEV_1 more than 20% predicted, pCO_2 < 7.3 kPa, upper lobe emphysema and a TLCO > 20% predicted.

In the case of a COPD exacerbation inhalers and oxygen therapy should be offered alongside oral prednisolone 30 mg for 7 to 14 days. Antibiotics are also appropriate comprising aminopenicillin, macrolides or tetracyclines.

Asthma

Aetiopathogenesis

Significant factors have been described. These include allergens such as the house hold dust mite and pets, viral infections particularly rhinovirus, tobacco smoke and pollutants. Additional factors of interest include sinusitis, obesity, GORD, drugs such as aspirin and NSAIDs, β Blockers and sprays/paints. Genetic studies have noted a strong association with CH13L1, IL6R, HLA DQ2 and SMAD3. The *hygiene hypothesis* is particularly relevant in asthma which explains a decrease in occurrence in those where exposure to environmental allergens early on helps to develop the immune system in its ability to protect against disease. This is why asthma is more prevalent in the Western world in view of its overall greater sanitation.

Asthma is deemed a T helper IgE allergic manifestation with CD4 T cells, eosinophils and mast cell build up. Th2 cells are responsible for the formation of IL4/5 and 13 which results in airway remodelling, hyper responsiveness, inflammation and smooth muscle hypertrophy/hyperplasia. Oedema and mucus plugging is noted along with fibrosis secondary to fibroblast activation. Mounting evidence suggests the occurrence of increased IL 25, 33 and Thymic stromal lymphopoietin resulting in natural killer cell, mast cell and eosinophil activation as well as the production of natural type 2 helper cells which further trigger lung inflammation.

Symptoms

Shortness of breath

Wheezing

Cough

Chest discomfort/tightness

Signs

Wheeze

Accessory muscle use

Differentials

Bronchitis

GORD

Pneumonia

Anaphylaxis

Investigations

Spirometry and peak flow measurements are valuable in the diagnosis of asthma. The following elements should be determined in the case of suspected asthma

- a large (>400 ml) response to bronchodilators
- a large (>400 ml) response to 30 mg oral prednisolone daily for 2 weeks
- serial peak flow measurements showing 20% or greater diurnal or day-to-day variability
- And return of the FEV_1 and FEV_1/FVC ratio to normal with drug therapy

Additional investigations of interest comprise fractionated exhaled nitric oxide which if positive implies evidence of eosinophilic inflammation and evidence for an increased probability of asthma. A positive skin prick test, increased serum eosinophilia >4% or a raised IgE to common aeroallergens also increases the probability of an asthma diagnosis.

Management

It is always important to note that preventative measures in asthma are essential. Initial steps include avoidance of provoking allergens as necessary. Certain foods, pets as well as the household dust mite are triggering elements. Smoking avoidance and weight reduction are valuable. In terms of medical treatment, a short acting β2 agonist is valuable in terms of short term relief. Inhaled steroids are the advisable drug of choice for prevention. They are recommended for those who use inhaled β2 agonists at least three times a week or more. Or who are symptomatic three times a week or more. Add on therapy comprises long acting β2 agonists or leukotriene receptor antagonists. If in the unfortunate event that symptoms still remain then patients should be provided increasing doses of inhaled steroids. Further therapies comprising a theophylline/tiotropium or slow release β2 agonist tablet should be offered. The final therapy of choice would be oral steroid tablets. It is important to also note that patients may suffer excessive steroid use which can be problematic. Hence therapies exist to help relieve overuse accordingly. This may include omalizumab given by injection (an anti IgE monoclonal antibody).

Acute asthma is of noteworthy mention at this point. Recognition of such deterioration is based on the following elements:

Acute severe asthma

Any one of: — PEF 33–50% best or predicted — respiratory rate ≥25/min — heart rate ≥110/min — inability to complete sentences in one breath

Life-threatening asthma

Any one of the following in a patient with severe asthma:

Clinical signs — Altered conscious level, Exhaustion, Arrhythmia, Hypotension, Cyanosis, Silent chest, Poor respiratory effort

Measured findings — PEF <33% best or predicted, SpO_2 <92%, PaO_2 <8 kPa, 'normal' $PaCO_2$ (4.6–6.0 kPa)

Near fatal asthma

Raised $PaCO_2$ and/or requiring mechanical ventilation with raised inflation pressures

Oxygen intervention is paramount in acute attacks with a saturation aim of 94–98%. Inhaled β_2 agonists are also of importance, typically nebulised, along with steroids as well as nebulised ipratropium bromide. IV magnesium sulphate as a single dose or infusion should be considered if there is no improvement in symptoms. It is important to note that such patients can deteriorate rapidly and discussion with ITU/HDU is recommended.

One of the most troublesome issues in asthmatic patients is inhaler technique and despite prescription it is known that those with asthma may not be utilising their inhalers adequately. Hence it is advisable to train patients accordingly in inhaler technique usage.

Occupational Asthma

At this point it is beneficial to discuss occupational asthma, a condition that occurs secondary to occupational agent exposure such as isocyanates, flour and grain, colophony and fluxes, latex, aldehydes, wood dust and animals. Typically patients describe an improvement in symptoms when away from work, on leave/rest days. It is important to note that atopy increases the risk of developing occupational asthma and that occupational rhinitis is a common co morbid occurrence. Investigations comprise peak flow measurements as well as skin prick and serological testing. Management relies on avoidance of high exposure work regions alongside the previously described treatment of asthma in general. However the symptoms and functional disturbance that occupational asthma induces can remain for a prolonged period despite avoidance. Individuals should undergo regular health monitoring (specifically serial PEF measurements) in order to detect early symptoms and signs of the condition. Under reporting of symptoms is common as workers may be concerned about risks to their employment status. Compensation can be sought in case of occupational asthma via the appropriate legal route.

Lung Cancer

Aetiopathogenesis

Two types of lung cancer exist; non small cell lung cancer and small cell lung cancer of which NSC is the most common. Tobacco smoke is a significant factor in relation to lung cancer. It is carcinogenic containing nicotine derived nitrosamine ketones and polyaromatic hydrocarbons which trigger DNA damage. Other factors of concern include asbestos exposure, pneumonitis, radiation exposure, pollutants, chromium, copper, beryllium, nickel, radon and arsenic to name but a few.

From a genetic standpoint, one observes activation of oncogenes such as Ras/c c-Myc Raf and inactivation of tumour suppressor genes such as p53 and retinoblastoma Rb. In NSCLC epidermal growth factor receptor mutations have been noted. There are various subdivisions of NSCLC which include adenocarcinoma, squamous cell carcinoma and large cell. Adenocarcinoma is seen most commonly in non smokers arising peripherally from bronchial mucosal glands; squamous cell is most associated with hypercalcemia and is seen centrally and large cell is the least prevalent, seen peripherally with evidence of focal necrosis.

Symptoms

Cough

Shortness of breath/difficulty in breathing (note that this can occur not only due to the tumour itself but due to involvement of the phrenic nerve and hence hemidiaphragm elevation)

Chest pain

Haemoptysis

Wheeze

Symptoms secondary to superior vena cava obstruction (facial swelling, headache, arm swelling, visual disturbance)

Hoarseness secondary to recurrent laryngeal nerve involvement

Dysphagia secondary to oesophageal compression effects

Symptoms secondary to Pancoast tumours leading to significant pain in the shoulder which spreads to the axilla/scapula due to involvement of the brachial plexus. Hand muscle discomfort may also occur

Bone discomfort secondary to malignant spread

Signs

Clubbing

Supraclavicular lymph node enlargement

Horner's syndrome, namely ipsilateral ptosis, miosis, enophthalmos and anhidrosis due to Pancoast tumour compression of the cervical sympathetic plexus

Signs of superior vena cava obstruction (distended neck veins, venous distension of the face and chest, facial oedema, upper limb oedema, papilloedema)

Reduced breath sounds and dullness on percussion in case of lung collapse

Signs secondary to a pleural effusion/pericardial effusion

Hepatomegaly secondary to malignant spread

Neurological signs secondary to brain or spinal cord involvement

It is important to be aware of paraneoplastic syndromes which can occur in non-small cell lung cancer but are more common in small cell. Manifestations arise from symptoms and signs attributed to hypercalcaemia due to excess parathyroid like hormone release, Syndrome of inappropriate antidiuretic hormone secretion and Cushing's syndrome due to excess ectopic Adrenocorticotropic hormone production, hypertrophic pulmonary osteoarthropathy (painful swollen joints), Trousseau's syndrome (migratory thrombophlebitis) and Lambert Eaton syndrome (proximal lower limb weakness > proximal upper limb weakness). Observe for hyperthyroidism in view of ectopic thyroid-stimulating hormone production and hypoglycaemia secondary to ectopic insulin like growth factor release. Cerebellar dysfunction can occur due to anti Yo or Purkinje cell antibodies. Poly and dermatomyositis may also be a finding.

Differentials

Pneumonia

Bronchitis

Pneumothorax

Pleural effusion

Tuberculosis

Investigations

An initial test of interest is sputum cytology particularly for centrally located tumours yet overall the diagnostic accuracy is limited. Blood investigations for paraneoplastic syndromes are advisable. Screen for elevated calcium levels, low serum sodium in view of SIADH (in addition to a serum osmolality < 280 mOsm/Kg and elevated urine osmolality) and disordered liver function in view of possible metastases. Imaging is key including a chest X ray for evidence of nodules/masses as well as pleural effusions. More advanced imaging includes CT scanning of the chest as well as of the abdomen and brain also in view of possible metastases. Bone spread can be assessed via skeletal scintigraphy. Positron emission tomography scanning can assist in nodule location and disease spread. Invasive tests include a bronchoscopy allowing visualisation of the tumour and biopsy sampling/bronchial brushings to be obtained. Ultrasound based thoracentesis allows pleural fluid to be sampled for assessment of malignant pathology. Thoracoscopy is a further diagnostic tool that can be employed if bronchoscopy proves futile. Mediastinoscopy can be useful for obtaining malignant tissue from within the mediastinum. It is important to note that staging of lung malignancy based on primary tumour, nodal involvement and spread is essential in subsequently guiding treatment. Hence investigations are employed to determine overall stage.

Management

Smoking should be ceased where applicable. Surgical intervention is advised for patients with NSCLC. Radiotherapy is also advisable for patients with stage I, II, III NSCLC. Chemoradiotherapy is the option of choice for patients with stage II/III NSCLC not suitable for surgery. Chemotherapy is advisable for patients with stage III/IV NSCLC. Suitable chemotherapy agents include docetaxel, gemcitabine, paclitaxel or vinorelbine in addition to a platinum drug.

Gefitinib is recommended for those patients with advanced or metastatic NSCLC with evidence of EGFR tyrosine kinase mutation positivity. Another EGFR TK specific chemotherapeutic agent is Erlotinib. Pemetrexed is advisable for NSCLC where no previous treatment has been received and the subtype is large cell or adenocarcinoma in nature.

For patients with small cell lung cancer cisplatin based chemotherapy is advised. Limited stage disease relies on chemo/chemoradiotherapy. Early stage SCLC relies on surgical intervention. Extensive stage SCLC benefits from platinum based chemotherapy. Oral topotecan has been recommended for those patients with relapsed small cell lung cancer.

For patients with endobronchial obstruction, it is advised to treat with radiotherapy and debulking or stenting. Effusions should be drained in addition to the use of talc pleurodesis. Opioids can assist to limit cough type symptoms. Stent insertion should also be provided to those with superior vena cava obstruction.

Disease spread to the brain should be managed with dexamethasone and radiotherapy. Bone metastases also benefit from radiotherapy intervention.

Mesothelioma

At this point it is worth highlighting the condition mesothelioma. Asbestos is the primary carcinogenic compound, and is noted in the following industries such as mining, ship building, insulation, ceramics and paper milling. Tumour suppressor gene involvement has been noted namely p16, p14 and NF2. Typically malignant mesothelioma should be suspected in those patients presenting with chest pain and evidence of pleural fluid and pleural thickening on chest X ray imaging. Further imaging relies on chest CT alongside CT/US guided pleural aspiration/ biopsy. PET scanning has been shown to assist in differentiating benign versus malignant disease states. Treatment focuses on early pleurodesis with talc for effusion management and indwelling pleural catheters if chemical treatment is unsuccessful. Surgical intervention is two fold, namely a pleurectomy with decortication and extrapleural pneumonectomy. Radiotherapy helps in the treatment of pain and breathlessness in case of superior vena cava obstruction. Chemotherapy namely pemetrexed and cisplatin have been shown to aid in symptom control and size reduction.

Pleural Effusion

Aetiopathogenesis

Pleural effusions occur secondary to a variety of mechanisms. These include impaired pleural membrane permeability, a reduction in intra-vascular oncotic pressure, increased capillary hydrostatic pressure, decreased lymphatic drainage and pleural space pressure reduction. Pleural effusions are either transudate or exudate in nature. Transudates tend to occur due to oncotic and hydrostatic pressure imbalance whereas exudates occur secondary to impaired lymphatic drainage and pleural inflammation. (A list of causes for either is further detailed under the examination section of pleural effusion).

Symptoms

Shortness of breath

Cough

Chest pain particularly worse on inspiration

Signs

Reduced chest expansion

Dullness to percussion

Reduced tactile fremitus

Reduced breath sounds

Mediastinal shift from the location of the effusion

Differentials

Pneumonia

TB

Lung malignancy

Congestive cardiac failure

Investigations

Imaging is beneficial in the first instance comprising a chest X ray. Pleural aspiration is advisable and should be screened for protein, lactate dehydrogenase, cytology, and microscopy/culture. Additional tests include a pleural pH (note a pH < 7.2 implies the need for chest drain insertion), glucose in case of suspected rheumatoid related effusions, TB culture, amylase for presumed pancreatitis pleural effusions, haematocrit for a diagnosis of a haemothorax and triglyceride/cholesterol level analysis to determine the existence of a chylothorax/pseudochylothorax.

Classification of an effusion is on the basis of Light's criteria which is as follows:

Pleural fluid is an exudate if one or more of the following criteria are met:

Pleural fluid protein divided by serum protein is >0.5

Pleural fluid lactate dehydrogenase (LDH) divided by serum LDH is >0.6

Pleural fluid LDH >2/3 the upper limits of the laboratory normal value for serum LDH

Additional investigations include a chest CT as well as MRI, although the latter is not routine. Furthermore one can consider a pleural biopsy where an effusion together with pleural nodules are noted and a thoracoscopy if initial pleural fluid aspiration proves non diagnostic.

Management

It is important to note that treatment of the underlying cause is advisable in cases of pleural effusion occurrence. By and large if patients are symptomatic with their effusions then insertion of a chest drain is recommended. In the case of malignant effusions, recurrence is common and consideration of a pleurodesis often with chemical talc is advised. Alternatives to talc as a sclerosant is bleomycin. If pleurodesis proves ineffective then the next option of choice is the insertion of an indwelling pleural catheter. In cases of a mesothelioma prophylactic radiotherapy should be offered at the site of drain insertion.

Pneumothorax

Aetiopathogenesis

There are numerous types of pneumothoraces. These are as follows:

A spontaneous pneumothorax is one that occurs following rupture of blebs or bullae in patients without underlying lung disease. An increase in shear forces are noted with associated lung inflammation and oxidative stress. A tension pneumothorax is associated with pleural damage with air inflow into the pleural space without outflow. Pressure subsequently rises with lung collapse and associated hypoxia. Causes of a tension pneumothorax comprise trauma which may be penetrating as well as bronchoscopy or barotrauma secondary to positive pressure ventilation.

Risk factors for a primary spontaneous pneumothorax include smoking, tall thin stature, pregnancy and Marfan's syndrome. A spontaneous pneumothorax can also occur secondary to COPD, asthma, TB, sarcoidosis, cystic fibrosis, pulmonary fibrosis, connective tissue associated lung disease, drug inhalation, pneumonia, lung malignancy and HIV associated Pneumocystis jirovecii pneumonia. A pneumothorax may be iatrogenic as a result of a lung biopsy, central venous catheter use, tracheostomy, intercostal nerve block or trauma.

Symptoms

Shortness of breath
Chest pain typically worse on inspiration

Signs

Tachypnoea

Asymmetrical chest expansion with tracheal shift to the contralateral
    side

Reduced breath sounds

Hyper resonate chest percussion

Reduced tactile fremitus

Differentials

Aortic dissection

Pericarditis

Acute coronary syndrome

Oesophageal rupture

Pulmonary embolism

Investigations

Initial investigations of choice comprise a chest X ray with consideration
of chest CT. Chest X ray findings comprise a linear shadow of pleura
with paucity of lung markings with evidence of a mediastinal shift.

Management

Management relies on size definition with a cut off of 2 cm. A pneumothorax greater than 2 cm between the lung margin and chest wall at the
point of the hilum defines a large as opposed to a small pneumothorax.
A small primary pneumothorax (PTX) without shortness of breath can
be simply observed. A symptomatic primary PTX or one that is > 2 cm
requires needle aspiration followed by a chest drain if unsuccessful.

　　If in the case of a secondary PTX patients require high flow oxygen
as well as chest drain insertion if > 2 cm or short of breath. If unresolved
then discussion with thoracic surgeons is needed. If surgery is unsuitable
then a chemical pleurodesis is advisable. For a secondary PTX less than
2 cm aspirate initially with subsequent drain insertion if unsuccessful.

TOPIC

Pulmonary Fibrosis

Aetiopathogenesis

Pulmonary fibrosis is an inflammatory condition initially which eventually leads to fibrosis. An initiating trigger may be smoking, viruses or aspiration based damage. There is associated cell death, increased permeability to proteins such as fibrinogen and the activation of epidermal growth factors which lead to proliferation. Matrix metalloproteinases cause basement membrane disruption via TGF β and continued fibroblastic activation occurs with further conversion of fibroblasts to myofibroblasts. Research has shown increased levels of prostaglandin E2 resulting in apoptotic resistance and hence persistent fibrotic changes. Genetic modifications are noted namely mucin 5B gene polymorphisms as well as caveolin 1. Furthermore mutations associated with telomerase have been described resulting in telomere shortening and hence impairing the lung repair process.

Symptoms
Cough
Shortness of breath (dyspnoea)
Fatigue
Joint discomfort (arthralgia)
Muscle discomfort (myalgia)

Signs
Bibasal crepitations which are fine inspiratory in nature

Clubbing

Evidence of pulmonary hypertension (such as a loud P2, tricuspid regurgitation)

Evidence of right ventricular hypertrophy (namely a right ventricular heave, an elevated JVP)

Differentials

Pneumonia (in the broadest sense could include, bacterial, fungal, viral)

Pneumonitis

Lung malignancy

Sarcoidosis

Investigations

Lung function, particularly transfer factor for carbon monoxide, is advisable in cases of suspected pulmonary fibrosis. If < 40% advanced disease is presumed. A decrease of > 10% in FVC or > 15% in TLCO of the initial 6–12 months implies a greater risk of mortality. Desaturation upon walking (at least 6 minutes) is also a common investigative measure. Imaging should rely on high resolution CT which will help to demonstrate reticular opacities and honey combing. Additional investigations of choice include bronchoalveolar lavage (BAL) and transbronchial lung biopsy (TBLB).

Management

Oxygenation will assist in terms of symptomatic issues along with pulmonary rehabilitation and opiates. Prednisolone (typically low dose) with azathioprine and N-acetylcysteine is recommended. Pirfenidone, a drug aimed at tapering fibrosis, has been recommended in those patients where their FVC ranges between 50–80% of what is expected. Consideration for transplantation should be made based on advanced disease namely TLCO < 40% predicted or progressive > 10% decline in FVC or > 15% decline in FVC during 6 months of follow up.

Pneumonia

Aetiopathogenesis

This section will focus primarily on bacterial acquired pneumonia. Hospital acquired pneumonia is highlighted under the examination section. Globally Streptococcus pneumoniae is the primary pathogen as well as Haemophilus influenzae, Mycoplasma, Legionella and Chlamydia. (Note: Viruses are also contributing organisms such as rhinovirus, influenza and coronaviruses.)

A bacterial pneumonia occurs following exposure to the organism in question as well as a reduction in the defence of the pulmonary system. One example of such is loss of upper airway reflexes allowing for organism entry into the lung. This may occur following CNS dysfunction or metabolic dysfunction. If the individual is already immunosuppressed with underlying pathology such as HIV or has chronic lung pathology (COPD) then the likelihood of susceptibility is greater. Virulence is a key feature of bacterial organisms. Consider Streptococcus pneumoniae and its associated Pneumolysin factor which aids in pulmonary tissue barrier dysfunction. Co infection with respiratory viruses can also further enhance the likelihood of bacterial infection. Viruses worsen the inflammatory condition and allow for greater bacterial adherence. Other factors of interest include smoking and dental hygiene issues such as periodontitis.

Symptoms

Cough productive in nature

Shortness of breath

Fever

Chest pain on inspiration

Signs

Evidence of sputum production. Note certain forms of pneumonia can lead to characteristic sputum patterns. For example Streptococcus is linked to rust coloured sputum and Pseudomonas can be linked to green coloured sputum.

Crepitations

Increased tactile fremitus

Evidence of a pleural effusion

There are a multitude of pneumonias. Two worth knowing well comprise Legionella and Mycoplasma.

Legionella pneumonia is often associated with exposure to air conditioning systems and contaminated water systems. Gastrointestinal features are seen such as diarrhoea, nausea and vomiting. An association with pancreatitis, hepatitis and SIADH is known.

Mycoplasma pneumonia is often seen in the young with a prolonged prodrome of fever, headache, diarrhoea and vomiting. Additional features include meningitis, encephalitis, neuropathy, myocarditis, pericarditis, joint discomfort, thrombocytopenia, disseminated intravascular coagulation, cold autoimmune haemolytic anaemia, erythema multiforme and erythema nodosum. An elevated IgM is often seen.

Other organisms of interest include

Staphylococcus aureus — notable in IV drug abusers

Klebsiella pneumoniae — seen in chronic alcoholics, COPD or diabetes

Chlamydia psittaci — secondary to bird handling

Coxiella burnetii — an atypical pneumonia that is responsible for Q fever. Sources of interest include sheep, goats, cats and cattle.

Differentials

Bronchitis
PE
Lung malignancy
Asthma
Pulmonary fibrosis

Investigations

Initial investigations of choice comprise a chest X ray as well as blood investigations which assess the white cell count for infection, CRP, liver function tests and urea and electrolytes. Sputum microscopy and culture as well as blood cultures are advisable. Urine screens can aid in the diagnosis of Streptococcus and Legionella. PCR of sputum samples can aid in the diagnosis of Mycoplasma.

Management

Oxygenation is advised ensuring a $pO_2 > 8$ kPa and saturation between 94–98%. The utilisation of antibiotics are key and are CURB 65 dependent.

- C confusion
- U urea > 7 mmol/l
- R respiratory rate > 30 breaths/minute
- B blood pressure < 90/60 mm Hg
- Age 65 or older

Low severity community acquired pneumonia relies on amoxicillin or doxycycline. Moderate severity (CURB65 2) centres on amoxicillin and clarithromycin orally or amoxicillin or benzylpenicillin and clarithromycin IV. High severity CAP i.e. CURB65 3–5 focuses on co amoxiclav and clarithromycin IV or benzylpenicillin in addition to levofloxacin or ciprofloxacin IV. Analgesia should be offered to those with pleuritic chest pain. Guidelines advise the utilisation of 5 days of antibiotics for low severity CAP with 7 to 10 days of antibiotics for those with moderate to high severity pathology.

It is worth mentioning the different treatments that exist depending on the type of pneumonia at this stage.

Streptococcus pneumoniae — Amoxicillin or Benzylpenicillin

Mycoplasma — Clarithromycin

Legionella — Fluoroquinolone

Pseudomonas — Ceftazidime and Gentamycin

Staphylococcus aureus — Flucloxacillin

Chlamydia psittaci — Doxycycline

Pulmonary Embolism

Aetiopathogenesis

Various risk factors have been described in association with the development of a PE. These include increasing age, prolonged travel, thrombophilia e.g. factor V leiden mutations which lead to protein C resistance or protein C/S/anti thrombin III deficiencies, obesity, smoking, hypertension, metabolic syndrome, trauma, post operative periods, oral contraceptives, pregnancy and malignancy.

Recalling earlier years at medical school you may remember Virchow's triad which comprises blood hypercoagulability, endothelial injury and stasis. These elements aid in thrombus formation.

Symptoms

Pleuritic chest pain
Shortness of breath

Signs

Tachypnoea/tachycardia
Hypotension
Cyanosis
Evidence of pulmonary hypertension with a loud P2, elevated JVP and
    tricuspid regurgitation

Differentials

Acute coronary syndrome

Pericarditis

Acute respiratory distress syndrome

COPD

Cardiogenic shock

Pneumonitis

Investigations

If one suspects a PE the Wells' score is advised for likely probability of such.

Clinical feature	Points
Clinical signs and symptoms of DVT (minimum of leg swelling and pain with palpation of the deep veins)	3
An alternative diagnosis is less likely than PE	3
Heart rate >100 beats per minute	1.5
Immobilisation for more than 3 days or surgery in the previous 4 weeks	1.5
Previous DVT/PE	1.5
Haemoptysis	1
Malignancy (on treatment, treated in the last 6 months, or palliative)	1

A score of 4 or more implies a PE is likely. The investigation of choice is a CT pulmonary angiogram. However in those where contrast is an issue and renal failure is present then a ventilation perfusion scan is advised. D dimer testing by and large has a limited diagnostic accuracy. It is useful in those patients with a minimum likelihood of a PE and if negative can be used to exclude the condition.

Management

Once a PE has been established the treatment of choice relies on low molecular weight heparin or fondaparinux. Patients with renal failure rely on the use of unfractionated heparin. For patients with evidence of haemodynamic dysfunction, management relies on thrombolytic intervention. Initial treatment should remain in place for at least 5 days until the INR reaches a threshold of 2 or more adjusted by a vitamin K antagonist. In patients with malignancy the treatment of choice is low molecular weight heparin for at least 6 months. A minimum of three months duration is required treatment wise once a vitamin K antagonist has been commenced extended if the event was unprovoked. Where anticoagulant treatment is hindered instigate the use of inferior vena cava filters. This is also true for those patients that suffer recurrent PE's.

Tuberculosis (TB)

Aetiopathogenesis

Various risk factors have been associated with TB infection. These include HIV, diabetes, malnutrition, overcrowded living environments, smoking, pollution, silicosis exposure, alcohol use, malignancy, end stage renal impairment, drug use such as anti TNF alpha agents and steroids. Various genetic abnormalities have been linked to the condition and include natural resistance-associated macrophage protein 1, interferon γ, nitric oxide synthase 2A, mannan binding lectin, vitamin D receptor, and some Toll-like receptors.

Mycobacterium tuberculosis is the primary pathogen of interest which is aerobic, acid fast and non motile and typically spread via droplet infection. Infection is first noted by detection of specific biochemical elements of the organisms such as N-glycolyl muramyl dipeptide which occurs courtesy of dendritic cells and macrophages. Neutrophils have been noted to respond through the production of antimicrobial peptides. T lymphocytes and macrophages respond to TB infection through the development of granulomas which helps on one hand to contain the infection but on the other hand allows the organism protection from further mechanisms of immune attack. Granulomas classically are viewed as central areas of caseous necrosis surrounded by epithelioid macrophages, giant cells and T lymphocytes along with surrounding fibrosis. In immune comprised individuals such as those with HIV infection, granulomas are not a common phenomenon.

Symptoms

Fever

Cough

Night sweats

Weight loss

Haemoptysis

Chest pain

Systemic symptoms e.g. neurological, genitourinary, skeletal, GI in case
of TB spread

Signs

Crepitations

Lymphadenopathy

Extrapulmonary signs e.g. neurological, chorioretinitis, cutaneous

Differentials

Bronchiectasis

Pericarditis

Aspergillosis

Lung malignancy

Investigations

Initial investigations of choice include the Mantoux tuberculin test with
purified protein derivative. The interferon gamma release assay for M.
tuberculosis is useful for the diagnosis of latent TB. Patients also require
HIV serology where TB is presumed. Sputum should also be obtained
for acid-fast bacilli smear and culture early in the morning and on three
consecutive days. Nucleic acid amplification tests are also advised for the
Mycobacterium tuberculosis complex. Imaging in the form of a chest X
ray is advantageous and can help to demonstrate evidence of consolidation, cavities, calcified nodules, or miliary TB where there are excessive

small nodular lesions present. In view of potential spread it is recommended that biopsy samples +/- fluid aspirates are taken accordingly e.g. lymph node, pericardium, pleura, bowel/liver/omentum/joint/bone marrow/urine (early morning)/cerebrospinal fluid/skin.

Management

Guidelines currently advise the utilisation of the following therapies in case of active TB without CNS involvement.

- isoniazid (with pyridoxine), rifampicin, pyrazinamide and ethambutol for 2 months **then**
- isoniazid (with pyridoxine) and rifampicin for a further 4 months.

Active TB of the CNS relies on the following regimen

- isoniazid (with pyridoxine), rifampicin, pyrazinamide and ethambutol for 2 months **then**
- isoniazid (with pyridoxine) and rifampicin for a further 10 months

TB of the central nervous system also relies on the use of steroids e.g. prednisolone or dexamethasone.

For those patients with evidence of multi drug resistant TB the recommended regimen is as follows

Drug resistance	First 2 months (initial phase)	Continue with (continuation phase)
Isoniazid	Rifampicin, pyrazinamide and ethambutol	Rifampicin and ethambutol for 7 months (up to 10 months for extensive disease)
Pyrazinamide	Rifampicin, isoniazid (with pyridoxine) and ethambutol	Rifampicin and isoniazid (with pyridoxine) for 7 months
Ethambutol	Rifampicin, isoniazid (with pyridoxine) and pyrazinamide	Rifampicin and isoniazid (with pyridoxine) for 4 months

In case of rifampicin resistance, patients should be offered a treatment protocol consisting of at least 6 drugs where sensitivity is likely. It is important to note in all cases of multidrug-resistant TB patients require hospital admission with the utilisation of a negative pressure room. Furthermore for any new diagnosis of TB, contact tracing is essential of close contacts.

Hypersensitivity Pneumonitis

Aetiopathogenesis

As the name suggests, this condition arises following antigenic exposure. The causes are numerous and can include chemicals eg isocyanates, animal proteins localised in fur, faeces or feathers, and microbes. One classic example is Bird fancier's lung secondary to inhalation of proteins located in birds' feathers and faecal matter. Another is Farmer's lung secondary to inhalation of hay dust or mould spores. By and large one observes an abundance of immunoglobulin deposition, proinflammatory cytokines, and complement. In chronic cases one observes an increase in Th1/ Th17 cells with production of IFN γ, TNF and IL 17/22. Overtime there is a shift towards a Th2 cell type and eventual fibrotic developments.

Symptoms

Cough
Fever
Chills
Shortness of breath
Headache

Signs

Fine bibasal crepitations
Fever
Clubbing
Muscle wasting

Differentials

Pneumonia

Sarcoidosis

Pulmonary fibrosis

TB

Asbestosis

Investigations

Initial blood investigations are advised comprising a full blood count, CRP and ESR. Sputum and bronchoalveolar lavage samples may help to identify precipitating antibodies that exist in reference to certain antigens. A chest X ray may help to demonstrate features of reticulonodular infiltrates as well as fibrotic developments. A high resolution CT helps to indicate ground glass opacities which are typically lower lobe based. Lung function tests can help to confirm disease with evidence of a restrictive pattern. Bronchoalveolar lavage may indicate the existence of neutrophils and lymphocytes. Additional findings may include mast cells, plasma cells and eosinophils. In addition IgA, M and G levels may be elevated.

Management

Treatment is typically of the underlying cause. Hence avoidance of the triggering antigen is paramount. If avoidance is not possible minimisation of exposure is needed either through protective equipment or environmental purification methods. Steroids typically prednisolone are recommended medical therapies with bronchodilators, sodium cromoglicate and anti histamine agents.

Obstructive Sleep Apnoea (OSA)

Aetiopathogenesis

OSA has been linked to craniofacial structural abnormalities and excess body fat resulting in increased pharyngeal airway collapse, poor upper airway muscle function along with respiratory control instability. There is also evidence to suggest the possibility of a reduction in lung volume overall in obese individuals and pharyngeal sensory impairment leading to upper airway collapse. Further concerns are the shift of fluid from the lower limbs to the neck region narrowing the pharyngeal airway. Men are at a greater risk of OSA and this has been attributed to the likely increase in central fat distribution and further lung volume reduction. An increased age has been linked to OSA with collagen damage and loss of the normal lung elastic recoil. Smoking is another risk factor assumed to cause OSA secondary to airway inflammation and impairment of sleep arousal thresholds which is also noted with an increasing age.

Symptoms

Regular Snoring
Breathing cessation typically witnessed
Gasping
Sleep disturbance
Daytime sleepiness
Headaches
Mood dysfunction

Memory disturbance

Sexual dysfunction

Nocturia

Signs

Increased neck circumference > 43 cm in men and 37 cm in women

Obesity

Enlarged tonsils

Pulmonary hypertension

Differentials

GORD

Hypothyroidism

COPD

Asthma

Narcolepsy

Investigations

The Epworth Sleepiness Scale should be used in patients with suspected sleep apnoea. A score of 10 along with excess daytime sleepiness, witnessed apnoea and excessive loud snoring strongly points to the diagnosis. Polysomnography is a further tool. Such studies demonstrate evidence of apnoea lasting 10 seconds or more with evidence of respiratory effort with a greater prevalence during rapid eye movement sleep. Additional investigations include the multiple sleep latency test which helps to more objectively assess sleepiness.

Management

Weight loss is the initial treatment of choice in OSA patients. Continuous positive airway pressure therapy based interventions are essential for moderate to severe conditions. For patients with evidence of respiratory failure, bi level ventilation is advised. Intra oral devices are also suitable for those patients who are unable to tolerate CPAP. Surgical intervention has been trialled but as yet is not widely recommended.

Aspergillosis

Aetiopathogenesis

Aspergillosis is associated with the Aspergillus hyphae which result in the production of metabolites which interfere with neutrophil and macrophage phagocytosis. Toll like receptors and dectin 1 receptors have the ability to recognise the pathogenic elements of Aspergillus and induce the maturation of antigen presenting cells with subsequent T cell activation. Various interleukins are produced, including IL4/5 and 13 which leads to the pathogenic response.

Symptoms

Productive cough mucous laden in nature
Haemoptysis

Signs

Fever
Wheeze

Differentials

Acute respiratory distress syndrome
Pneumonia
Bronchiectasis
TB
Sarcoidosis
Hypersensitivity pneumonitis

Investigations

Initial investigations of choice comprise assessing for the existence of eosinophilia, skin prick testing for Aspergillus fumigatus, determining the presence of asthma, elevated IgE levels (typically > 1000 IU/dl) as well as elevated IgG and A levels in the case of possible allergic bronchopulmonary aspergillosis. Sputum testing for aspergillus is also recommended. Imaging should be undertaken and includes a chest X ray which helps to indicate fleeting infiltrates or evidence of atelectasis in the case of ABPA. The presence of an aspergilloma is seen as a mass typically upper lobe based. For the diagnosis of invasive disease a bronchoscopy together with BAL is useful.

Management

Primary treatment is medical with the utilisation of steroids namely prednisolone as well as anti fungal treatment such as itraconazole. There is also evidence to suggest the benefits for the utilisation of omalizumab, an anti IgE agent. If in the case of an aspergilloma, resolution may occur through the utilisation of itraconazole or amphotericin. However surgical resection is preferred depending on patient suitability. Bronchial artery embolization for severe haemoptysis is an option of worth.

In terms of prophylaxis, anti fungal agents such as fluconazole, itraconazole and voriconazole are effective as well as amphotericin.

Pulmonary Hypertension

Aetiopathogenesis

Pulmonary hypertension (PH) is associated with a mean arterial pressure > 25 mm Hg at rest or > 30 mm Hg during exercise based activities. Numerous causes exist including genetic such as ALK2 gene mutations, drugs such as fenfluramine, an anorectic, which has now been withdrawn, collagen vascular diseases, thromboembolism, chronic lung disease, left sided heart dysfunction, haematological disorders and metabolic disorders. PH can also be idiopathic in nature.

Symptoms

Shortness of breath on exertion

Fatigue

Chest pain

Syncope

Cough

Right sided abdominal pain

Signs

Loud P2

Systolic murmur lower left of sternum most commonly (tricuspid
    regurgitation)

Pulmonary regurgitation

Elevated JVP

Hepatomegaly

Palpable ventricular heave

Differentials

Aortic stenosis

COPD

Cardiomyopathy

Obstructive sleep apnoea

Hepatic failure

Restrictive lung disease

Investigations

Initial investigations comprise a full blood screen with an arterial blood gas to help in the assessment of hypoxia. Six minute walk testing should be employed. Chest X ray imaging helps in the detection of enlarged pulmonary arteries. ECHO assessment helps to detect valvular abnormalities along with right ventricular/atrial dilation and increased pressures. A Doppler ECHO helps to estimate pulmonary artery pressure (PAP).

A ventilation perfusion scan helps to exclude the presence of thromboembolic disease. Pulmonary function testing is advised. If in the case of difficulties with Doppler ECHO use, right sided cardiac catheterisation is employed to better determine pulmonary artery pressure.

Management

Treatment in the first instance can rely on the use of anti coagulants in case of thromboembolic occurrence, diuretics such as frusemide to aid in oedema relief, oxygenation, and vasodilators such as calcium channel blocks to help minimise pulmonary vascular resistance.

Lung and heart lung transplantation should be employed in advanced stage disease (New York Heart Association III/IV) where patients remain symptomatic and the disease continues to progress. Additional medication of value is as follows:

Prostaglandins — e.g. epoprostenolol or iloprost. Side effects of such drug agents comprise flushing, headaches, jaw pain, diarrhoea and nausea.

Endothelin receptor antagonists — e.g. bosentan. Side effects of such drug agents include flushing and syncope. Liver dysfunction may also occur.

Phosphodiesterase inhibitors — e.g. sildenafil. Side effects comprise flushing, headaches, diarrhoea and muscle aches.

Bronchiectasis

Aetiopathogenesis

Bronchiectasis is classically an inflammatory disorder with neutrophil and T cell prevalence and associated cytokines such as IL 8 and TNF alpha. Numerous causes exist and these can include infectious agents such as Mycobacterium or Klebsiella, Aspergillus or viruses, namely influenza, congenital disorders such as cystic fibrosis, primary ciliary dyskinesia or alpha 1 antitrypsin deficiency, immunodeficiency either primary in nature (hypogammaglobulinemia) or secondary to malignancy, rheumatological disorders, foreign body inhalation, gas exposure such as chlorine/ammonia, bronchial obstruction or inflammatory bowel disease.

Symptoms

Cough
Mucous laden sputum
Pleuritic chest pain
Fever
Weight loss

Signs

Crepitations
Clubbing
Wheeze
Ronchi (low pitched rattling)

Differentials

Alpha 1 Antitrypsin deficiency
Asthma
COPD
Pneumonia
Cystic fibrosis
TB

Investigations

Initial blood investigations comprise serum immunoglobulins namely IgG/A and M and serum electrophoresis. Patients should also undergo screening for antibody deficiencies. Exclusion testing for the presence of CF is recommended alongside ciliary function testing in cases where chronic upper respiratory tract infections are common. Imaging in the form of a chest X ray but primarily a high resolution CT is advisable. Bronchial wall dilation and thickening are evident features. A signet ring appearance is often typically described. Sputum sampling for microscopy culture and sensitivity is recommended. Lung function testing is also recommended which typically demonstrates an obstructive picture. A restrictive pattern is seen in advanced stages, particularly with the occurrence of fibrosis and atelectasis.

Management

Patients should be mentored and managed in reference to appropriate airway clearance intervention, with relevant breathing techniques and postural drainage along with forced expiration techniques. Sterile water inhalation is also beneficial along with nebulised saline. Antibiotic intervention is valuable. Discussion with microbiologists at your local hospital trust should be undertaken to help guide the process. Initially sputum should be sent for culture and sensitivity means. First line antibiotic treatment comprises amoxicillin or clarithromycin. If patients are colonised with Pseudomonas aeruginosa then ciprofloxacin should be commenced. Haemophilus requires amoxicillin for those with chronic colonisation. Individuals with more than three exacerbations a year require long term antibiotic therapy. If despite medical therapy there is no improvement in symptomatology the most appropriate intervention at this point would be surgical with lung resection as the primary treatment option.

TOPIC

Sarcoidosis

Aetiopathogenesis

Researchers suggest that sarcoidosis is predominantly an excessive immune based response to partially degraded mycobacteria and pro-pionibacteria, specifically PAMPS (pathogen associated molecular patterns). In acute sarcoidosis there is an increase in CD14 positive macrophages with an increased TNF alpha response. Further cytokines of interest include IL 2 (courtesy of CD4 T cells), and interferon gamma. Th17 cells have been reported with a decreased production of T regulatory cells. Formation of non necrotising granulomas occurs over time. Genetic associations include HLA DRB1 03/14/15.

Symptoms

Cough
Shortness of breath
Joint pain
Haemoptysis
Fatigue
Depression

Signs

Crepitations
Oxygen desaturation on exertion
Lupus pernio
Bilateral uveitis
Arrhythmias

Cranial nerve dysfunction

Evidence of hypothalamic/pituitary disturbance

It is important to note the existence of Lofgren's syndrome — an acute form of sarcoid associated with erythema nodosum, polyarthritis and bilateral hilar lymphadenopathy.

Differentials

Pneumonitis

Lung cancer

TB

Investigations

Initial blood investigations may demonstrate an elevated serum amyloid A or angiotensin converting enzyme. Hypercalcaemia is also noted. Liver dysfunction can occur hence liver function screening is paramount in particular serum alkaline phosphatase. Imaging in the form of a chest X ray helps to demonstrate the feature of bilateral hilar lymphadenopathy and infiltrates with evidence of fibrosis towards end stage disease.

Note the staging of X ray findings namely:

Stage 0 — normal

Stage 1 — bilateral hilar lymphadenopathy (BHL)

Stage 2 — BHL and infiltration

Stage 3 — infiltration

Stage 4 — fibrotic change

An HRCT can help to further define the presence of alveolitis or fibrosis. An ECG can help to determine the presence of arrhythmias, or bundle branch block. In view of hypothalamic pituitary dysfunction patients should be screened for evidence of diabetes insipidus and hyper prolactinaemia in the first instance. Pulmonary function testing will confirm typically a restrictive pattern along with a decrease in diffusing capacity of the lungs for carbon monoxide. Histological assessment via biopsy helps to confirm the diagnosis. This can be achieved via bronchoscopy usually endobronchially. Non necrotising granulomas are characteristic. Induced sputum assessment helps to ascertain the CD4: CD8 ratio with an elevation helping to exclude non granulomatous lung disease.

Management

Treatment relies on the utilisation of steroids with bisphosphonates to ensure protection against steroid induced osteoporosis. Alternatives to steroid treatment include methotrexate and azathioprine. Anti-malarial agents namely chloroquine and hydroxychloroquine are beneficial in the management of skin lesions as well as bone dysfunction and neurological related complications. Infliximab is another agent of choice particularly useful for skin dysfunction.

Surgical intervention is employed in advanced stage sarcoidosis and comprises primarily of lung transplantation.

Cystic Fibrosis

Aetiopathogenesis

Cystic fibrosis (CF) is an autosomal recessive disease and occurs secondary to a genetic mutation in the Cystic fibrosis transmembrane conductance regulator channel which impairs chloride and bicarbonate transport. This results in reduced or impaired anion transport, mucous abnormalities with increased viscosity and lung injury. There is also associated hyperinflammation and excess sodium reabsorption, reduced airway surface liquid hydration and impaired muco ciliary clearance. Mutations of CFTR are numerous and are typically missense in nature, the most prevalent being Phe508del. Frameshift and splicing can also occur.

Symptoms

Cough

Wheeze

Shortness of breath

Meconium ileus in neonates with associated nausea, vomiting and
    abdominal pain/distension

Steatorrhea

Purulent sputum

Signs

Nasal polyps

Rhinitis

Signs of respiratory distress

Wheeze

Crepitations
Clubbing
Hepato splenomegaly
Evidence of intestinal obstruction
Postural disturbance eg kyphosis/scoliosis
Evidence of malabsorption/failure to thrive
Undescended testicles/hydrocele

Differentials

Sinusitis
Bronchiectasis
Asthma
Aspergillosis

Investigations

Diagnosis of CF relies on the demonstration of a sweat chloride greater than 59 mmol/L and/or two CF causing CFTR mutations in trans, alongside sputum cultures positive for Pseudomonas aeruginosa, exocrine pancreatic insufficiency, salt loss syndrome and obstructive azoospermia in case of male gender. It is important to note that sputum testing may also localise Haemophilus influenzae, Staphylococcus aureus and Burkholderia cepacia as additional organisms. Two CF causing mutations are deemed diagnostic in view of the autosomal recessive nature of the condition. Additional tests of interest comprise evidence of pancreatic insufficiency via faecal elastase testing or ion channel involvements. Imaging in the form of a chest X ray will confirm the presence of pulmonary nodules, infiltration and hyperinflation. An abdominal X ray will demonstrate dilated loops of bowel in case of meconium ileus. Contrast barium enema is also useful in this regard. Lung function testing will in essence demonstrate an obstructive picture in such patients. Further testing can rely on measurement of immunoreactive trypsinogen which is typically elevated in CF presenting in neonates.

Management

Treatment of Pseudomonas aeruginosa infection is essential. This can be achieved via tobramycin, colistin and ciprofloxacin. Azithromycin can aid in limiting chronic infection. Chest physiotherapy is recommended to aid in airway clearance. Mucolytics such as dornase alfa is advisable. Hypertonic saline along with mannitol are preferred lung hydration agents. Currently research is underway to develop more specific drug agents aimed at CFTR modulation. One such agent is Ivacaftor useful in those patients with the G551D mutation. Appropriate nutritional intervention is advisable with regular monitoring accordingly. Pancreatic enzyme supplements are a must in view of insufficiency. Patients should be screened for CF related diabetes and managed with insulin accordingly. Liver dysfunction such as cirrhosis along with biliary disease such as cholelithiasis should be managed appropriately. Bone dysfunction can be best treated with bisphosphonates and vitamin D/calcium supplementation. Further complications such as constipation, bacterial overgrowth and GORD also require addressing. End stage lung disease requires transplantation and the following criteria aid in such intervention:

- FEV1 < 30 percent predicted
- Oxygen therapy assistance
- Hypercapnia
- Frequent exacerbations and prolonged antibiotic use
- Worsening symptoms particularly among the young

Surgical intervention is also relied upon as an intervention for CF related complications such as nasal polyps, pneumothorax and rectal prolapse.

Examination Skills

Introduction

Effective examination skills are key to determining a diagnosis along-side an accurate history. During medical school and early junior doctor years the assessment of examination skills during an OSCE or post-graduate examination setting is something feared by most, if not all. Regardless of this fact it is important to note that there are only a finite number of stations that can appear. What you must remember is that the mark schemes at either an undergraduate/postgraduate level are universal. Examiners are expecting you to demonstrate an appropriate rapport with the patient in the first instance being mindful of any concerns they may have during the examination. In addition, candidates should be able to perform a thorough and systematic systems examination and be prepared to detect physical signs, construct differentials and detail potential investigation and management strategies. Each station is schema dependent, so be weary of preferred presentation style. For example, an examiner may simply ask you to palpate the abdomen. In addition some may prefer you not to talk through your examination as you perform it. You can imagine how laborious it becomes for them when the candidate begins as follows: 'I am standing at the end of the bed and observing for any scars or masses… I am now looking at the hands for clubbing etc etc…' It may seem that they are rushing you through but that is so they can reach all station aspects and ensure you can gain as many points as possible.

The following cases are all likely at an undergraduate and postgraduate level, some harder than others. However if faced with difficulty keep things simple and DO NOT invent signs. Examiners are quick to spot the actor type candidate and this will not bode well in terms of professionalism/probity. Be observant of the fact that you are only likely to face a two to three minute interplay with the examiner post examination so follow the pattern of signs, differentials, investigations and management and make sure to keep it sharp and most of all simple. Examiners get frustrated with long drawn out negatives and several random causes which are not applicable to pathology in the UK. In other words an opening discussion could be something along the following lines... 'On examination the patient appears comfortable/distressed. There is evidence of x, y and z. The most likely diagnosis is... secondary to x, y and z.'

Or

'I am unsure of the diagnosis but would like to offer the following differentials. In order to obtain a diagnosis I would undertake the following tests.'

Start with blood investigations before imaging. And if you are 100% convinced of the diagnosis then offer a management plan. OK, on to the cases!

COPD

Patients with COPD in an OSCE are likely to be stable in their condition. Note the presence of audible wheeze and prolonged expiration. Hands wise there is likely to be evidence of nicotine discolouration and potential asterixis in case of CO_2 retention (unlikely in an exam setting!). Observe for accessory muscle use and an over inflated chest. During chest percussion patients will have evidence of hyper resonance and on auscultation there will be an audible wheeze predominant during expiration. Observe generally for utilisation of inhalers, nebulisers and oxygen therapy. Additional bonus points may arise from being able to demonstrate evidence of pulmonary hypertension secondary to COPD. This will be evident via possibly a loud P2, elevated JVP and tricuspid regurgitation. Patients with COPD are also often regular users of steroids so the astute candidate will be able to determine whether there is evidence of such use, namely myopathy, bruising and a Cushingoid appearance.

The differentials, investigations and management have been described previously in this text. Common examiner questions may focus specifically on the acute management of the condition and the indications for surgical intervention. Examiners may also open up a broad discussion on respiratory failure. Two types exist as follows:

Type 1 — hypoxia is the predominant feature. Causes comprise COPD, PE, ARDS, pneumothorax, pneumonia, pulmonary oedema, asthma, bronchiectasis, pulmonary fibrosis, kyphoscoliosis, obesity, pulmonary artery hypertension, congenital cyanotic heart disease

Type 2 — characterised by hypoxia and hypercapnia. Classically seen in severe asthma, worsening COPD, drug overdose, neurological dysfunction such as head and cervical cord dysfunction, poly neuropathy, muscle dysfunction, Myasthenia gravis, obesity, hypoventilation syndrome.

Be aware of the term Chronic hypercapnic respiratory failure — associated with bicarbonate production to compensate for hypercapnia, occurring over a several plus day period. Hence only a minimal decrease in pH is noticed.

Investigations should focus on attempting to determine the underlying cause with regular arterial blood gas sampling, imaging, pulmonary function testing and echocardiography. Management relies on hypoxia/ hypercapnia correction with appropriate ventilator support and correction of the underlying cause.

A discussion may commence regarding ARDS. The following criteria comprises the condition: an initiating clinical condition (e.g. sepsis, burns) — acute onset — bilateral infiltrates documented by chest radiograph at end-inspiratory position — pulmonary artery wedge pressure $\leq$ 18 mmHg and/or absence of clinical evidence of left atrial hypertension — PaO_2/FiO_2 ratio $\leq$ 200 in a stable state after the patient has adapted to standardised ventilation.

Additional aetiological factors comprise trauma, fractures, pneumonia, aspiration, drug overdose and drowning to name but a few. Patho physiologically there is associated epithelial and endothelial damage with increased pulmonary permeability. Management relies on assisted ventilation with lower tidal volumes and sufficient Positive end-expiratory pressure allows reduced mortality along with prone positioning. The use of steroids, prostaglandins and nitric oxide have been described but have not demonstrated sufficient survival benefits.

Type II respiratory failure in view of its coexisting hypoxia and hypercapnia can provoke discussion. Guidelines recommend Non-Invasive Ventilation with an oxygen saturation between 88–92 percent. NIV commencement should occur with a pH < 7.35 and pCO_2 > 6.5. Absolute contraindications to NIV use include facial burns, upper air obstruction and facial trauma. If NIV fails to stabilise CO_2 with a likely risk of respiratory arrest then immediate referral to intensive care is warranted. A full knowledge of NIV settings in relation to pathology is not necessary. One of interest is COPD where recommended initial NIV settings comprise an IPAP of 15 and EPAP of 3.

Pulmonary Fibrosis

In the examination of a patient with pulmonary fibrosis, the initial step (like with all respiratory examinations), is to determine the degree of breathlessness at rest. Observe for oxygen utilisation and a cough. Typically the cough will be non productive. Examine for evidence of steroid use, namely bruising, Cushingoid appearance and proximal myopathy. Cyanosis and clubbing may be present and chest expansion may be limited. Percussion is typically dull basally with fine end inspiratory crepitations on auscultation, again typically basally. Fullness to the examination relies on assessment of associated conditions. This may include examining for rheumatological phenomena, namely arthropathy, nodules, telangiectasia, sclerodactyly, Raynaud's phenomenon and a butterfly skin rash. In the case of dermatomyositis observe for Gottron's papules or a heliotropic rash peri orbitally. There may be lordosis or kyphosis in case of ankylosing spondylitis or café au lait developments in neurofibromatosis. Observe also for features of sarcoidosis as highlighted earlier. The investigations, differentials and management of pulmonary fibrosis have been described already. Examiners may inquire about the possible causes of apical and basal fibrosis more broadly. Apical fibrosis is typically seen in Extrinsic Allergic Alveolitis, Allergic bronchopulmonary aspergillosis, Sarcoidosis and radiation along with TB, Ankylosing spondylitis, Silicosis and Coal worker's pneumoconiosis. Basal fibrosis is seen in idiopathic pulmonary fibrosis, connective tissue disease and asbestosis.

Pulmonary Consolidation

Consolidation is typically diagnostic of pneumonia. Observe for a productive cough, reduced chest expansion, dullness on percussion and increased vocal resonance (note consolidation leads to an increase in vocal resonance versus an effusion where resonance is decreased). On auscultation you will typically observe crepitations which are coarse in nature. The examiner may prompt you for other causes of consolidation in general and this may be malignant or embolic related. The differentials, investigations and management of pneumonia have been previously described. Pay close attention to the CURB 65 criteria as this pinpoints assessment severity and treatment accordingly.

It is important to note that pneumonia may also be hospital acquired and examiners may probe in this regard. Such a condition arises in 48 hours post hospital admission. Organisms include Staphylococcus aureus, Gram negative organisms such as Klebsiella and Pseudomonas and fungi. Aspiration pneumonia is also a feature of those patients with neurological compromise such as a stroke or decreasing Glasgow Coma Scale. Anaerobic organisms predominantly result in this condition. Treatment of hospital acquired pneumonia relies on imaging, blood and sputum cultures and discussion with in hospital microbiology for the optimum treatment of choice depending on what is localised.

Examiners may also probe for the causes of cavitating pneumonia and this comprises Staphylococcus aureus, Klebsiella, Pseudomonas, TB and Aspergilloma.

Bronchiectasis

In such patients observe for evidence of a productive cough, with finger clubbing. There is typically no dysfunction of chest expansion with resonant percussion (however in cases of associated fibrosis chest expansion will be reduced and there will be dullness on percussion) as well as inspiratory crepitations which are coarse on auscultation. Note that such crepitations can alter with coughing and there may also be an expiratory wheeze. There may also be an inspiratory click heard without the need for a stethoscope. The differentials, investigations and management have been described previously.

Examiners particularly like to focus on the causes of bronchiectasis and so be sure to recall these. Examples include childhood infections e.g. pertussis, measles, bronchial obstruction e.g. tumour or foreign body, pulmonary fibrosis, ciliary clearance dysfunction e.g. cystic fibrosis, immotile cilia syndrome, Allergic bronchopulmonary aspergillosis and autoimmune disease e.g. IBD and rheumatoid arthritis, as well as congenital anatomical defects.

Pleural Effusion

The classic signs for a pleural effusion on examination are reduced chest expansion, dullness to percussion described as stony dull with reduced air entry on auscultation together with reduced vocal resonance. If the effusion is significant one will note tracheal deviation to the opposite side. For this station sound knowledge of the causes of a pleural effusion are needed. Ensure an understanding of the causes of an exudate and transudate.

Exudate — protein > 30 g/l. Examples include malignancy (lung being the obvious one along with lymphoma, leukaemia, breast, ovarian, GI), infection such as pneumonia or TB, connective tissue dysfunction such as systemic lupus erythematosus or Rheumatoid arthritis, PE, asbestosis, sarcoidosis, drugs e.g. bromocriptine, methotrexate, nitrofurantoin.

Transudate — protein < 30 g/l. Examples include cardiac failure, pericarditis, nephrotic syndrome, cirrhosis, hypothyroidism, hypoalbuminaemia.

A sound knowledge of causes therefore aids in determining additional signs. In the case of malignancy examine for lymphadenopathy. Observe for arthropathy or a butterfly skin rash in case of connective tissue disease. Cardiac failure will be associated with an elevated JVP, oedema and a 3rd/ 4th heart sound. Hypoalbuminaemia is often linked to evidence of poor nutrition and oedema. Make sure to recall well the Light's criteria along with the differentials, investigations and management of a pleural effusion described earlier.

Lung Cancer

This is likely to be one of the most extensive cases during a clinical examination in view of the signs associated. The general status of the patient is highly important observing for evidence of malnutrition and muscle wasting. Note evidence of nicotine staining and clubbing. Hypertrophic pulmonary osteoarthropathy may be evident depicted as tender and swollen joints in the hands, elbows, knees and ankles. Hoarseness may occur with involvement of the recurrent laryngeal nerve. Muscle wasting of the hands may be seen due to Pancoast tumour occurrence and associated nerve root damage, namely C8-T1. A further consequence of Pancoast tumour would be Horner's syndrome and the triad of ptosis, miosis and anhidrosis. Observe and examine astutely for lymphadenopathy paying attention to any neck vein distention/enlargement as well as an oedematous face and upper limbs which would signify superior vena cava obstruction. Depending on the associated pathology there may be tracheal deviation. If in the case of a pleural effusion this may involve tracheal deviation to the opposite side and if in the case of collapse this would involve deviation towards the area of collapse. Collapse/effusion would lead to diminished breath sounds and dullness on percussion along with reduced chest expansion. Observe for scars which could indicate previous lung resection. In case of lung resection, either a lobectomy or pneumonectomy, observe for reduced chest expansion, tracheal deviation to the area of resection, dullness to percussion and reduced breath sounds in case of a lobectomy with absent breath sounds in case of a pneumonectomy. Note inward drawing of the ribs as well. If probed further on collapse in general remember the typical causes. These include (bar lung cancer), COPD, bronchiectasis, asthma, sarcoidosis, trauma, effusion, pneumothorax and TB to name but a few.

The differentials, investigations and management have been highlighted above. Examiners often ask about paraneoplastic states of lung cancer so it is advisable to know this aspect well. A detailed understanding of lung cancer staging will be highly unlikely to be questioned.

Previous TB

This case is unlikely to be a common occurrence during undergraduate examinations. However it has been included for completion. In this case there is likely to be an overlap of findings. This may include evidence of apical fibrosis (dullness to percussion, reduced chest expansion, apical inspiratory crepitations), or thoracoplasty which is marked by noticeable rib resection. A thoracoplasty was one of the earliest methods to treat TB where rib removal led to collapse of the lung with the aim to allow it to heal with rest. Be mindful of a left supraclavicular scar indicating a phrenicotomy (phrenic nerve crush) which allowed for paralysis of the diaphragm and elevation of the lung aiding healing.

Examiners may inquire about other previous methods of treatment which included the occurrence of artificial pneumothoraces to allow the affected lung to collapse and hence recover as well as postural rest where patients would be instructed to lie on the diseased side to inhibit lung movement and encourage organ rest. There was also the use of artificial weights (up to 5 pounds) placed on the clavicles to limit lung movement and induce rest.

Imaging

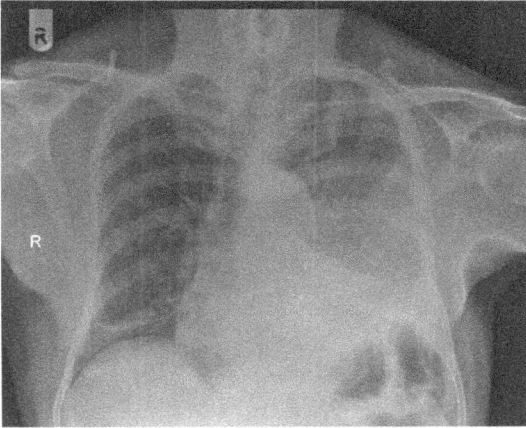

Fig. 10.   Evidence of left lower lobe consolidation and pleural effusion

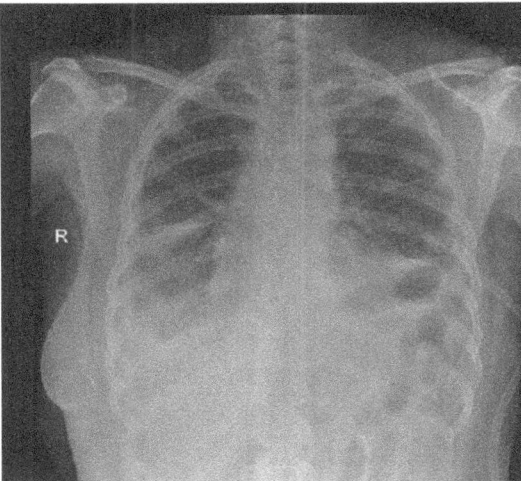

Fig. 11.   Bilateral pleural effusions

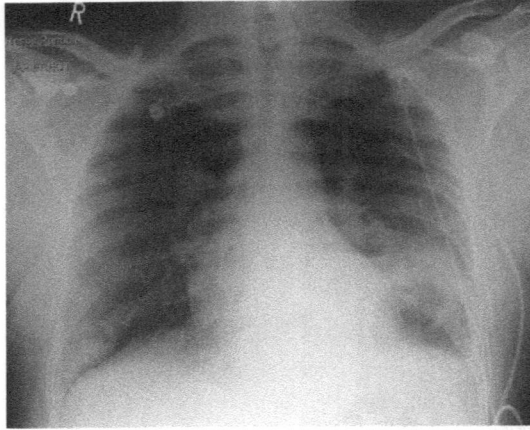

Fig. 12.   Cavitating lesions in a patient with pneumonia

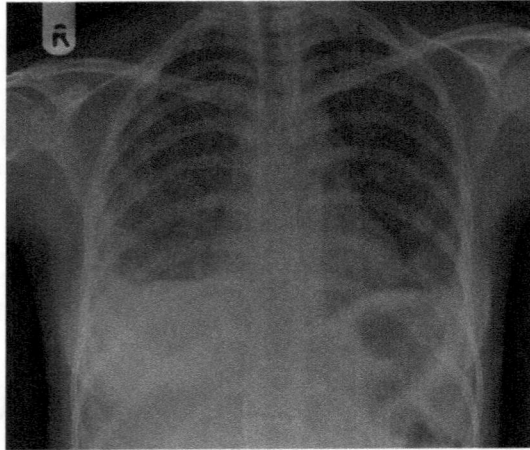

Fig. 13.   Miliary opacifications in keeping with miliary TB

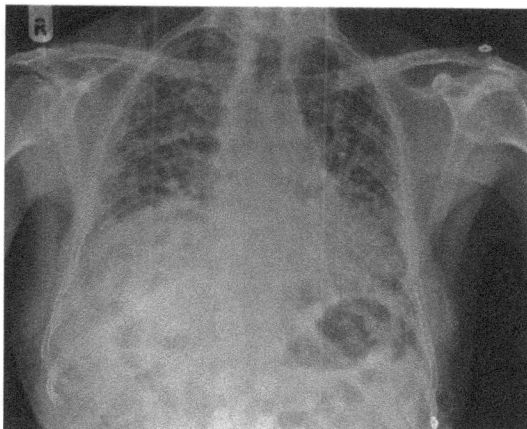

Fig. 14.   Evidence of pulmonary fibrosis

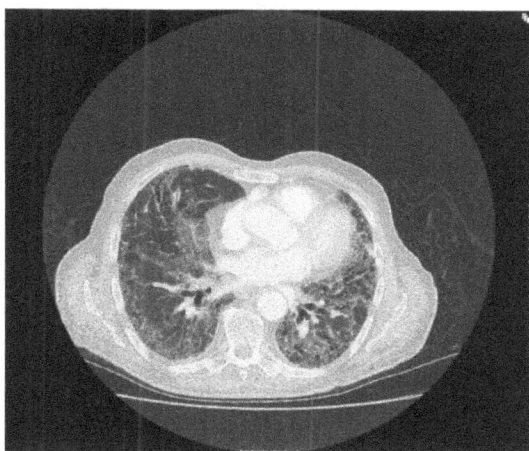

Fig. 15.   High resolution CT demonstrating evidence of honey combing and reticular opacities in pulmonary fibrosis

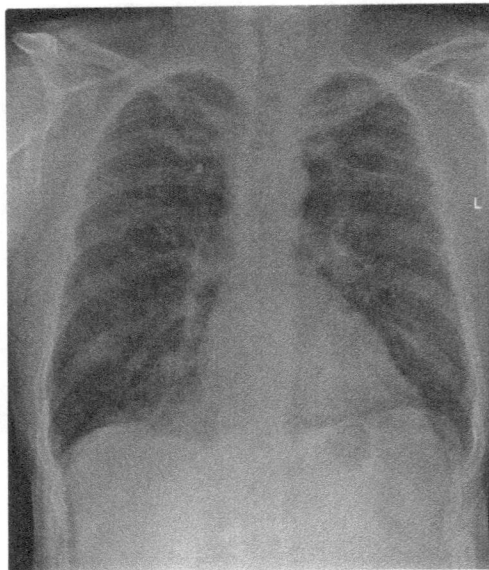

Fig. 16.   Classic chest X ray of a patient with COPD. Note the hyperinflated lungs and bullae in the left upper zone

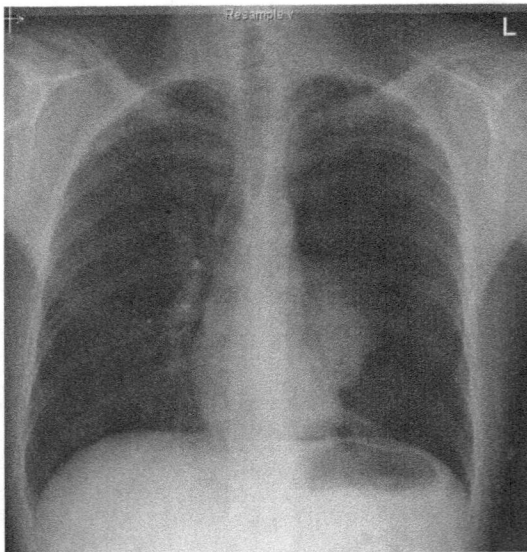

Fig. 17.   Left sided pneumothorax

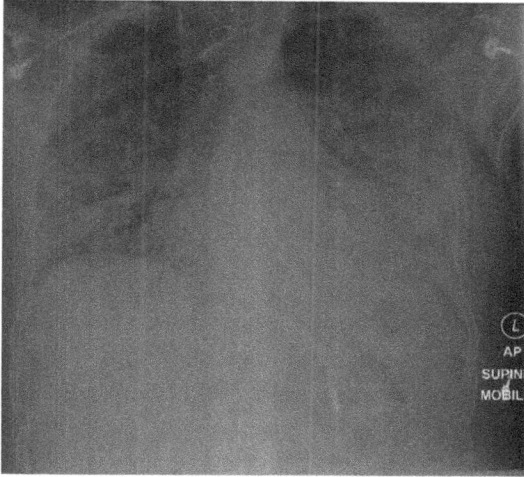

Fig. 18.   Bilateral reticulonodular infiltration in keeping with extrinsic allergic alveolitis (hypersensitivity pneumonitis)

References

Annotated BTS Guideline for the Management of CAP in Adults. Available from
https://www.brit-thoracic.org.uk/document-library/clinical-information/
pneumonia/adult-pneumonia/annotated-bts-cap-guideline-summary-of-
recommendations/

Appraisal of the Drug Treatments Used in Pulmonary Arterial Hypertension
(PH). Available from https://www.nice.org.uk/guidance/gid-tag382/documents/
pulmonary-arterial-hypertension-association-uk4

Barker AF. Bronchiectasis. *N Engl J Med* 2002;346:1383–1393, doi: 10.1056/
NEJMra012519.

British Guidelines on the Management of Asthma. Available from https://www.
brit-thoracic.org.uk/document-library/clinical-information/asthma/btssign-
asthma-guideline-2016/

BTS Guideline for Interstitial Lung Disease Guideline. Available from https://
www.brit-thoracic.org.uk/standards-of-care/guidelines/bts-guideline-for-
interstitial-lung-disease-guideline/

BTS Pleural Disease Guideline. Available from https://www.brit-thoracic.org.
uk/document-library/clinical-information/pleural-disease/pleural-disease-
guidelines-2010/pleural-disease-guideline/

Chronic Obstructive Pulmonary Disease in Over 16s: Diagnosis and Management.
Available from https://www.nice.org.uk/guidance/cg101/resources/chronic-
obstructive-pulmonary-disease-in-over-16s-diagnosis-and-management-
35109323931589

Clinical Investigation of Medicinal Products in the Treatment of Patients with
Acute Respiratory Distress Syndrome. Available from http://www.ema.
europa.eu/docs/en_GB/document_library/Scientific_guideline/2009/09/
WC500003553.pdf

Decramer M *et al*. Chronic obstructive pulmonary disease. *Lancet* 2012;
379(9823):1341–1351.

Goldhaber SZ *et al*. Pulmonary embolism and deep vein thrombosis. *Lancet* 2012;379(9828):1835–1846.

Guideline for Non CF Bronchiectasis. Available from https://www.brit-thoracic. org.uk/document-library/clinical-information/bronchiectasis/bts-guideline-for-non-cf-bronchiectasis/

Guidelines for the Ventilatory Management of Acute Hypercapnic Respiratory Failure in Adults. Available from https://www.brit-thoracic.org.uk/ document-library/clinical-information/acute-hypercapnic-respiratory-failure/bts-guidelines-for-ventilatory-management-of-ahrf/

King TE *et al*. Idiopathic pulmonary fibrosis. *Lancet* 378(9807):1949–1961.

Lawn SD *et al*. Tuberculosis. *Lancet* 2011;378(9785):57–72.

Lung Cancer Diagnosis and Management. Available from https://www.nice. org.uk/guidance/cg121/resources/lung-cancerdiagnosis-and-management-35109444863941

Management of OSA in Adults. Available from http://www.lothianrespiratorymcn. scot.nhs.uk/wp-content/uploads/2010/11/SIGN-73-Management-of-Obstructive-Sleep-Apnoea_Hypopnoea-Syndrome-in-Adults.pdf

Martinez FD *et al*. Asthma. *Lancet* 2013;382(9901):1360–1372.

O'Sullivan BP *et al*. Cystic fibrosis. *Lancet* 2009;373(9678):1891–1904.

Segal BH. Aspergillosis. *N Engl J Med* 2009;360:1870–1884, doi: 10.1056/ NEJMra0808853.

Smyth AR. *et al*. European Cystic Fibrosis Society Standards of Care: Best Practice guidelines. *J Cyst Fibros* 2014;13:S23–S42.

Tuberculosis. Available from https://www.nice.org.uk/guidance/ng33/chapter/ recommendations

Valeyre D *et al*. Sarcoidosis. *Lancet* 2014;383(9923):1155–1167.

Venous Thromboembolic Diseases: Diagnosis, Management and Thrombophilia Testing. Available from https://www.nice.org.uk/guidance/cg144/chapter/ recommendations

Disclaimer

This text was produced in reference to current guidelines. At the time of publication there may have been further updates to the evidence and the reader is advised to be aware of this fact. Furthermore any drugs listed may or may not have drug dosages listed to minimise potential errors. Readers are advised to refer to the latest pharmaceutical formularies for clarification.

Notes

Index